Preface

The Figtree Food Program is based on a wise approach to food that I was gifted to stumble on over 25 years ago. At the time I was desperate to find strong healing supports, having just been discharged from conventional treatment for lymphatic cancer after exhausting all known treatment protocols. The reins were placed back in my hands, which, after the initial shock, proved to be a powerful wake-up call. I felt I had no choice but to face this challenge head-on and become deeply involved in my own healing process, with the great hope of finding ways to influence the course of my life.

Through intensive searching, several influences emerged, one of which was a naturopathic doctor who advised me on a nutritional program that I committed myself to wholeheartedly. It was powerful, as were the other modalities I was involved with during this time — visualization and meditation — and they worked, against the odds. I survived and healed and, as the story many times goes, eventually began to share my experience with others in need, especially in regard to nutrition.

Eventually I became a nutritional health practitioner, and was able to witness a wide variety of health challenges responding to the same basic nutritional support that had so profoundly affected my health. At one point the realization occurred to me that if children could be taught this commonsense approach to supporting their well-being, they could avoid the degenerative conditions that increasingly plague our society — conditions such as obesity, diabetes, digestive problems, asthma, allergies, heart disease, arthritis, and even cancer. With that insight, the seed of this book took root.

May *Eat Smarter* encourage greater awareness, greater health, and greater happiness to all who read it.

from their parents. *Eat Smarter* shows the best way to help children, and to help parents help their children, gain the health and appearance they deserve for a lifetime.

John McDougall, M.D.
www.dmcdougall.com
March 1992

Introduction

For many years I have been deeply aware of the critical need for children and teenagers to better understand how their food habits affect their health and appearance. As a nutritionist, I try to do whatever I can to spread helpful, relevant nutritional information in this direction. My opportunity to do so, in the form of a book, came together after the advent of a new person in my life — a stepson named James.

James was a sweet-natured, smart and funny 10-year-old. He was also a junk-food addict who was beginning to get a little pudgy. My nutritional background set the stage for us squabbling at each meal about his poor food choices, and consequently our relationship was often frustrating for both of us. Before my eyes, James was growing increasingly larger — not because of the usual growth spurts, but due to serious weight gain. Finally though, I gave up nagging and accepted him as he was, realizing that enjoying our time together was much more important to me than having food issues taint our friendship.

As time passed, James continued to expand into a very overweight teenager. Sadly his sweet personality was also changing, becoming negative and bullying. I remember one time, while driving in the car, hearing James murmur under his breath from the back seat how his legs were turning into huge tree trunks.

Nevertheless, he was resistant to changing his food habits until, at age 14, he spent the summer with his dad and me on the Spanish island of Mallorca. The first day we went swimming, James refused to take off his shirt, too ashamed to be seen in a bathing suit, and referring to himself as a "beached whale."

After two weeks of torment, James had had enough. He approached us, asking for help. We were overjoyed with this opportunity, but I knew we had to proceed carefully and cleverly, for it would probably be our one big chance to make a difference.

To start, I made many of James's favorite foods, but upgraded them with healthier ingredients. I made sure there were always healthy treats in the house so James never felt deprived, especially when he knew his friends were eating ice cream and candy. I have to admit we were not above using bribery, as James's father promised to buy him a pair of fancy sport shoes at the end of the summer if he stuck to the food program.

We approached this challenge creatively and tried to make it fun. By the end of the summer, not only had James stuck to the program but, to our delight, he actually enjoyed it. One of the things we did was create different food adventures. For example, we staged a "blind taste test" where we blindfolded James and then fed him a variety of foods, some of which were new to him and some he thought he disliked. Surprisingly, James discovered he actually liked more foods than he realized.

As we explored new tastes and recipes, I would explain to James how each food benefited the health and balance of his body. It was important to him to understand why some foods were good for him, and others were not. This worked better than simply giving him a list of "dos and don'ts."

At the end of the summer, James went back to England where he lived with his mom. By that time, he was two sizes smaller, had more energy, felt a lot better about himself, and was proudly wearing his new pair of shoes. His mom was overjoyed to make the same wholesome foods for both of them.

Four months later, when James came back to visit for the holidays, his dad and I were amazed. He had become a lanky, handsome teenager. Not only was his sweet personality back, but there was more. James was empowered and felt really good about himself by seeing how he could affect his health, his shape, and his life. The experience gave him a strong sense of self-confidence, which was more than we had anticipated, and a gift to us all.

James is now 26 years old. He is healthy and physically fit, and is working towards becoming a professional writer. In addition, he has created a successful business working with food — as a personal cook for several top movie stars while they are filming on location. The work is demanding, but for James it is also a pleasure. There is no doubt that the seeds planted when he was 14 have sprouted well and flourished.

The experience with James helped me educate other children and teens, as well as their parents. In my work as a nutritionist, I often encountered ill and out-of-shape people stuck in poor eating habits they had developed as children. In spite of their condition, they still chose unhealthy foods that, in many cases, were slowly killing them. I came to realize that it is much easier to change course at an earlier age, before poor food habits become permanent.

With this in mind, I have created two books in one. The first part of *Eat Smarter: The Figtree Food Program* is for parents, adults and teens. Its focus is the simple cause-and-effect relationship between our food choices, good health, and health challenges. Toward this end, I have included a section on creating a healthful and effective food plan, plus many simple and delicious recipes.

The second part of *Eat Smarter, James' Story*, is a storybook for kids. Youngsters are inquisitive and want to know how things work, especially if that information is presented in a way that is fun and easy to grasp. This is true for the child in all of us that

too often remains in control of many of the decisions we make
— especially in regard to food.

Although the storybook is simplified, it incorporates a con-
densed version of "The Basics of Nutrition," a course I taught to
graduate students. My hope is that by offering knowledge and
deeper understanding, children as well as teens and adults will
be encouraged and empowered to take pride in making food
choices that lead to feeling great and looking good!

Medical Supervisions Page

If you are ill or on medications, do not attempt this food program without the supervision of a physician experienced in the effects of dietary changes.

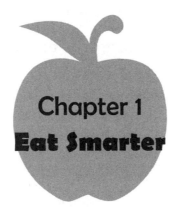

Chapter 1
Eat Smarter

For children to thrive and develop into healthy, balanced, competent adults, the role nutrition plays is far more important than most people realize. Good nutrition is not only vital to health, normal body weight and shape, clear skin, easy digestion, and high energy, but it is also a relevant factor in concentration, balanced temperament, self-esteem, and even intelligence. In order to provide children with a strong foundation of health and well-being and encourage a healthy relationship with food, it is essential to teach them to cultivate good eating habits — the earlier the better.

Through my years as a nutritional health practitioner, I have discovered that presenting children and teens with simple, clear and interesting information about food engages their natural curiosity about wanting to know the way things work. Relevant nutritional information about what food truly is, what it does in our body, its relationship with health and disease, and how to make choices that support looking good and feeling vibrant, opens the mind and senses to exploring and discovering new tastes and creating new conditioning — based on common-sense and understanding, as well as enjoyment.

For parents, what is required is a deeper understanding of the food they are offering their children and its effect in the body. A little imagination is needed in upgrading old favorite recipes and discovering newer, healthier ones. Since children learn mostly by example and observation, parents may need to upgrade their own eating habits. The early years, when parents have control over their child's food choices — usually up until a child begins school — are an extremely valuable time in which to instill a strong foundation of healthy food habits. Once children mix with their peers, it may seem that all the good conditioning is out the window, as extreme-tasting, adulterated foods become freely accessible. But I have witnessed that sooner or later early conditioning seeps back in, and children actually find pride in choosing tasty foods that are also good for them.

The big question these days is, just what constitutes healthy food habits? It can be confusing, with fad diets continually circulating, and clever, deceptive advertising by big food manufacturers attempting to hypnotize people into believing that poor-quality food is actually good for them. On top of this, health professionals can have widely differing opinions from one another. For everything you read or hear, the opposite perspective is available to completely confuse the issue. What is a parent to do? The only thing that I've witnessed works long-term is that which is tried and true, not complicated, and leaves plenty of room for innovative expression. Presented in a delicious and creative way, this is what the Figtree Food Program is all about.

Chapter 2
The Figtree Food Program

It's never too late, or even too early, to open to a new level of awareness regarding wise food choices. Releasing old habits that are detrimental to our health can be an inner struggle between those parts of us in charge of food choices. Is it the child who is hankering for treats and rewards, or a frustrated part of us that yearns for comfort, or the intelligent bright part that responds to that which makes the most sense? We all contain those three voices and more — yet it is always within our field of choice to commit ourselves to selecting one way, creating the support, and gathering the information needed to keep our decision on track. In that spirit of making intelligent and wise choices, the Figtree Food Program presents a way of eating and understanding food and food choices that is delicious and satisfying, as well as healthy.

It is important to understand, right from the start, that the Figtree Food Program is not a fad diet, but rather a common-sense way of eating based on the profound effects of an abundant variety of high-nutrient foods on the body. This exceptional program was not created by me, but was shared with me at a time of great personal need, and it literally transformed my body. During my nutritional practice of 20 years, I have watched the program transform many people's health — children and adults alike. This way of eating has a tradition that goes back through history — with the Natural Hygiene practitioners in the early 1800s, all the way back to Hippocrates, who proclaimed that food should be our medicine, and medicine, our food.

When abundant raw materials and energy are available, the body will initiate its self-healing programming to its fullest potential. The innate ability of our highly intelligent bodies to self-heal, repair, balance, regenerate, and adjust to a healthful weight is beyond what most people imagine is possible. This is where food choices come in.

The Standard American Diet (S.A.D.) is much too high in empty calories (according to statistics on the current epidemic of obese children and adults), and far too low in nutrients, such as vitamins, minerals, essential fatty acids, and enzymes. With minimal nutrients, people barely have enough needed nutritional support to get through the day, which is why there is a strong urge to grab a coffee, a soda, something sweet — anything to give a jolt. It also means there are not enough nutrient-based raw materials left over at the end of the day to be used in needed deep repair and regenerative work, and therefore many degenerative conditions, such as pre-diabetes and pre-arthritis, continue to progress and eventually develop into disease.

On the other hand, when a person consumes meals full of a variety of high-nutrient foods, there are usually more nutrients, rather than more calories, taken in than are needed to get through the day. With extra calories, there follows extra weight. But when there are extra, quality raw materials, the body uses them for background work, which translates into repair, regeneration, and adjusting body weight. When extra nutrients are available day after day, the body has more freedom to address any area of sluggishness, stored waste, and unhealthy, weakened or irritated tissues. The cells are then able to do their best job at repairing and restoring balance to every part of the body. Most degenerative conditions —arthritis, diabetes, clogged arteries, hormone imbalances, acne, and so on — can self-heal. These are not diseases of germs and bacteria — they are degenerative conditions created primarily by a build-up of waste, toxicity or irritation. Abundant amounts of high-nutrient foods also stimulate the metabolism to function at higher levels, and excess weight melts away.

Chapter 3
A New Perspective on Weight Loss

When it comes to children or teens carrying excess weight, it is much easier for them to readjust their weight and metabolism rate during the early years, before repeated dieting takes its toll. Each time a person diets, they lose equal amounts of protein and fat. But when weight is put back on, usually more fat is regained than protein, meaning that the fat-to-protein ratio becomes lopsided — more fat and less protein in the tissues. Eventually the fat-to-protein ratio ends up so out of balance that excess weight becomes very difficult to reduce.

The bottom line about dieting is that ultimately, "Diets don't work!" The view that in order to lose weight, people need to eat less — less calories, less food — is the opposite of what truly works. The Figtree Food Program's approach is instead about encouraging people to eat greater quantities of wholesome foods, high in nutrients, and therefore producing long-lasting, healthful weight.

Common Misperceptions on Dieting

If weight loss is attempted through reducing food intake (reducing nutrients as well as calories), the body will ultimately feel depleted and deprived. Reacting as if in a famine, the body will respond by slowing down metabolism — a self-preservation mechanism that reduces the rate at which cells burn nutrients for fuel. Weight loss then levels out and literally gets stuck, becoming more difficult to shift, while food cravings intensify — the exact opposite result dieters are hoping for.

Attempting to lose weight on a "high-protein" fad diet while greatly reducing foods high in carbohydrates creates other problems, since the body's first choice of fuel is always carbohydrates. They are the most plentiful type of food on the planet, are easily turned into energy, and burn cleaner than fat or protein, which are usually only turned into fuel when carbohydrates are not available. If you deprive the body of carbohydrates in order to lose weight, it will crave them and eventually create an imbalanced metabolism where carbohydrates are burned slower due to their scarcity.

On top of that, heavy protein intake can put a strain on the kidneys. Also, since proteins are actually acids — amino acids, to be exact — a diet of more than 60 grams of protein daily presents a lot of acid for the body to neutralize. And the main neutralizing substance that is used for this purpose is calcium. Therefore, high-protein diets can lead to calcium depletion, especially from the bones.   Another problem with a high-protein diet is that much of the protein usually comes from animal products containing too much cholesterol and saturated fat. These types of fat contribute to clogged arteries — the number one killer in this country — as well as to inflammatory diseases, such as arthritis and cancer.

Also, a great misunderstanding about high-protein diets is that they list certain carbohydrate-rich foods —potatoes, yams, carrots, fruit, and whole grains — as problem foods, because they are high on the glucose index — the rate at which glucose (that is, carbohydrates) gets into the bloodstream. This is a shortsighted misperception and is not the whole picture of how food is used in the body. These types of whole foods are nutrient-rich and provide the body with many benefits. Potatoes, for example, are rich in potassium, vitamin C, and even some protein. If potatoes are combined with a large amount of fresh vegetables, the resulting healthy meal will not contribute to weight gain. Instead, it will raise the body's nutrient levels and help flush out toxins and waste due to its strong fiber and high-water content. The real problem with carbohydrates has to do with refined and processed carbohydrate-rich foods — such as sugar, sodas, pasta, breads and popular cereals — that have been stripped of their nutrients. Many people don't realize that foods like these contribute more to excess weight gain than even fatty foods. When a refined carbohydrate food is eaten, because of the lack of fiber that normally regulates the flow of glucose from the carbohydrate into the bloodstream, a sugar spike occurs. Too much glucose enters the bloodstream all at once, and places a heavy demand on the pancreas to produce large amounts of insulin to pull glucose into the cells. Such continual harsh demands on the pancreas can lead to diabetes.

On top of that, a glucose spike in the blood means too much fuel is available — more than the body can use at that time. The mechanisms of the body are such that the extra glucose cannot just sit around in the bloodstream waiting to be used, so whatever is not immediately used for fuel gets stored in fat deposits for future use, which translates into weight gain.

Long-Term Healthy Body Weight

The trick to weight loss is really no trick at all. The body wants to be at its most healthy weight. Because high levels of nutrients stimulate the body's metabolism to work at a higher rate, the body can and will adjust its weight — without dieting on reduced calories. It is important to understand that the higher the nutrient base, the more the metabolism is stimulated. More energy is then available to clear out excess weight, as well as waste and toxicity, and make repairs where needed. And, because the body will not feel deprived, as it does with dieting, the chances of maintaining a healthier weight are much greater. For people who are underweight, this same system of consuming plentiful quantities of high-nutrient foods will healthfully increase their weight. In the end, it is the strong nutrient base that allows the body to adjust to its healthiest state.

Exercise is also an important catalyst for increasing metabolism, but if it is pushed when there are not enough nutrients available (as occurs with reduced food intake diets), the body will become even more depleted. Then metabolism will slow down, and the body will be more vulnerable to exercise-related injuries and illnesses.

The bottom line for the Figtree Food Program approach to weight loss is: YOU CAN BURN OFF EXCESS WEIGHT WHILE BECOMING HEALTHIER.

Chapter 4
The Figtree Food Program for Kids of All Ages

When discussing foods that support health as well as weight adjustment and regeneration, it is important to understand that foods do not directly heal or change us. Food, as it is found in nature, is actually an exquisitely designed package of quality nutrients. Food provides raw materials for the body, but does not possess the intelligence to act on the body. It is the body's cells that act on the food, appropriating the raw materials to fuel the body's work. The more quality raw materials available, the more freedom and potency the body has to perform repair, readjust its weight, and regenerate itself wherever needed.

Good nutrition for children and teens encompasses the same basic cellular needs — a strong, balanced nutrient intake. Of course, there is a greater need for protein and calories at growth spurts, and more of certain vitamins at different stages of development, but the truth of the matter is, if you present three meals daily consisting of generous quantities of high-nutrient foods, the nutritional needs of children and teens will be more than met. A strong balanced nutrient intake translates into meals that contain a generous combination of seven essential nutrients: carbohydrates, fats, proteins, vitamins, minerals, fiber, and water. All-natural, unadulterated (unchanged from its original state) foods grown on the earth contain all seven nutrients, but each food has a unique combination of these seven. Some foods have more protein, some more carbohydrates, while others have higher fat content, and others, higher water content.

• Foods that contain high levels of wholesome *carbohydrates* are fresh fruits and vegetables, whole grains, beans, potatoes and yams.

• Foods that contain high levels of *protein* are nuts and seeds, soy, beans, many whole grains, fish, poultry, dairy products, and meat. Foods such as beans and grains contain strong quantities of *both protein and carbohydrates*, and low quantities of fat.

• Healthy *fats* are most concentrated in avocados, olives, nuts and seeds.

• *Vitamins* and *minerals* are rich in all unadulterated plant foods. In order for plants to stand upright and produce fruit or vegetables, these nutrients must be present. If soil is organic and cultivated without chemical fertilizers, the vitamin and nutrient levels are usually even higher.

• All unprocessed vegetable and non-animal foods contain *fiber*, an important material that helps move food through the digestive tract, absorbs and carries excess fat and toxins out of the body, and regulates the even absorption of nutrients into the bloodstream. Animal products do not contain any fiber; therefore, when consuming them, it is important to eat fiber-filled vegetable foods at the same time.

• The *water* contained in natural foods is very valuable to the body, and is much higher quality than bottled water. High-water-content foods, such as vegetables and fruits, contribute plentiful water for the body's tissues, help move food through the digestive tract with ease, and contribute to the flushing out of wastes and toxins. Eating a higher percentage of drier concentrated foods, like bread, power bars, and meat, and then drinking bottled water does not create the same favorable conditions for the digestive tract as consuming meals full of high-water-content foods.

To insure strong nutrient support, foods need to be prepared in ways that don't destroy their rich vitamin, mineral or fiber content, while at the same time are still attractive and taste good. When foods are processed or changed, they begin to lose some of their initial nutrients — the more processing, the greater the loss of nutrients. Whole-wheat kernels, for instance, are abundant in B vitamins, minerals and fiber, but by the time they end up as pasta, there are almost zero nutrients left except for empty concentrated calories. The same is true with brown rice versus white rice, and especially so with sugar.

Raw, unadulterated foods contain the highest amount of vitamins and minerals, along with live enzymes that are added to our body's own supply of digestive enzymes. When raw food is heated above 110 degrees, live enzymes are destroyed. Therefore, to ensure we get live enzymes and high levels of vitamins and minerals, it is wise to eat at least one fresh raw food in every meal. When cooking, to retain as many nutrients as possible, it is best to steam or bake food. Sauteing quickly in a little olive oil is next best. Deep frying and boiling both destroy the greatest amounts of nutrients. If fried food is eaten in a restaurant, chances are that it is cooked in unhealthy oils. The healthiest oil to use for cooking, dressings and sauces is cold-pressed, extra-virgin olive oil. It is best bought in a glass container, as oils can leach toxic chemicals from plastic bottles.

Dealing with Food Quantities

As youngsters go through growth spurts, their needs for more all-round nutrients increases, not just for protein, as most people think. This translates into needing to eat larger quantities of food, plus more snacks. Determining the correct quantities of food for different ages and stages of growth differs vastly when dealing with processed, refined foods as compared to whole foods.

In processing and refining foods, when the original fiber, water, and vitamin and mineral content are removed or destroyed, the calories become more concentrated. Therefore, concentrated-calorie foods usually contain many more calories compared to the exact same quantity of the same whole food before it undergoes processing. Smaller amounts of processed food can have higher amounts of calories, making it easy to overeat.

If too much concentrated-calorie food is consumed, the body will have to deal with more calories than it can actually use for fuel at any one time. As mentioned earlier, since the body has learned through the ages never to get rid of possible fuel in case of a famine or a long cold winter, it will convert the extra calories into stored fat. There is almost an unlimited amount of extra fat the body can store.

On the other hand, when whole foods are presented at meals, there is usually no need to restrict calories, since the bulk (fiber and water) in these foods fill one up before too many calories are consumed. This allows children, teens, and even adults to eat until their innate sense of fullness clicks in and they feel satisfied.

Therefore, when choosing foods for meals and snacks, processed, refined, concentrated-calorie food recipes should be either converted to healthier food by upgrading the ingredients, or should be eliminated or consumed infrequently.

Processed, Refined, Concentrated-Calorie Foods

Common foods in this category are: sugar; white flour products found in pasta, pizza flour, cereals, breads, rolls, cakes, cookies and crackers; white rice; sodas; most candy; breakfast bars; chips; fruit juices; jams; jello; high-fructose corn syrup; ice cream; and alcohol.

Besides contributing to weight problems, studies show that a high intake of processed, concentrated-calorie foods creates a dramatic increase in childhood health challenges, such as diabetes, allergies, intestinal problems (such as bad breath, excess gas, belching, and stomach aches), Attention Deficit Disorder (ADD), and teenage acne.

Irritating or Toxic Foods

Even more problematic for children and teens are substances that are toxic or irritating to the body.

• *Trans fats* (hydrogenated and partially hydrogenated fats) — found in margarine and many baked goods, including chips, cookies, cakes, frozen entrees, and many other foods — are unlike any fat found in the body. Studies suggest they may damage the cell's DNA and contribute to heart disease, cancer, and other degenerative diseases.

• *Canola oil* is a genetically altered toxic rapeseed oil that was created in Canada, hence the name. Studies suggest that low levels of toxicity from rapeseed are still present in canola oil and create DNA damage in lab animals.

Canola oil has turned up in many health foods, since it is an inexpensive monounsaturated oil with no taste.

• *Chemicals* added to foods, such as preservatives, colorants, and emulsifiers, along with pesticide residues, may irritate and poison cells. Many of these in use in the U.S. have been banned in other countries that consider them potentially toxic.

• *Artificial sweeteners*, such as aspartame and saccharine, are linked to cancer in lab animals, as well as to brain disorders.

• *Commercial fried foods* are generally fried in rancid and/or unhealthy fats that create free radicals and damage cells.

• *Commercial animal products* —meat, poultry, eggs, and dairy products that contain added hormones (to fatten animals or force them to overproduce) — are now being linked to increased risks of hormonal cancers and premature puberty.

High-Allergenic Foods

The following group of foods may contribute to the allergies and asthma that have become increasingly common in children.

• *Dairy products* are among the highest allergy-producing foods. Studies link dairy products to excess phlegm, ear infections, upper respiratory infections, and gastric distress.

• *Wheat products* are considered high-allergy-producing foods.

• *Sugar and chemical food additives* have been related to allergic reactions that contribute to Attention Deficit Disorder, hyperactivity, and poor concentration in children and adults.

Unfortunately, a high percentage of these problematic foods are served at school, as well as masterfully advertised on TV, especially for kids' programs. By educating ourselves, through our consumer power we can upgrade the food choices that are available to us and our children.

Chapter 5
The Figtree Food Program Meal Plan

The most important thing about a quality food program is not only eating food that is good for you, but also enjoying the taste of the food and feeling satisfied afterwards, not hungry or deprived.

Getting a child to try new foods can be challenging. Becoming a bit of a trickster has its benefits. Making new foods for yourself and nonchalantly asking your child if they want a taste or even better, to help in the cooking, can sometimes be more successful than direct force. Also, making their favorite foods in an upgraded version with healthier ingredients can be a major first step in higher-nutrient meals. An example would be spaghetti with pasta sauce. Instead, you could make spaghetti squash, which after cooking produces long pasta-like strands. Added to this could be a tomato pasta sauce with many vegetables, such as zucchini, string beans, carrots and chard. If these are foods your child refuses to eat, simply blend them into the tomato sauce, and no one will know but you that you've produced a high-nutrient meal.

The following menus are full of tasty, easy-to-make, high-energy, high-nutrient foods. It is important to eat generous portions of these foods at each meal in order to increase the body's nutrient base and stimulate metabolism. Most of the foods on this program are low-and medium-calorie, so that the few high-calorie foods included are balanced.

High-Nutrient Breakfast Choices

Just the word – "break [the] fast" — says a lot. After eight hours of not eating, most of the body's water-soluble vitamins and minerals are low, and energy foods are in reserve. This is the time, especially for kids and teens, to consume a plentiful amount of nutrients to set the foundation for the day. The morning's nutrient base also sets the metabolism — will the body have abundant fuel and raw materials and therefore available energy, or will it need to slow things down in order to make do on too little?

The American way has been to start breakfast with orange juice. Fruit sugar from fruit juice gets into the bloodstream too quickly, and some fruit sugar will end up as stored fat, just as with white sugar. Instead, I suggest eating fresh cut-up fruit, as the fiber in the fruit will better regulate the fruit sugar's absorption into the blood, ensuring it will all be used for fuel. Alternatively, if the juice is made not from fruit but from fresh vegetables that contain less natural sugar, the morning juice becomes more like a powerful vitamin and mineral drink, and an excellent way to start the day.

Juice Blasters

Carrot Celery Juice
Mixed Veggie Juice
Lemon Flush

High-Powered Breakfast Choices

Fresh Fruit Ambrosia with Chopped Nut Topping
Creamy Cinnamon Oatmeal Cooked with Fruit
Veggie Avocado Omelet with Salsa
Banana Walnut Pancakes (my favorite)
Muesli with Fresh Fruit, Seeds, and Banana Almond Milk
Millet Waffles
Scrambled Tofu

High-Nutrient Lunch Choices

When we consider lunch, the sandwich has become the midday standard. Looking more closely, the nutrients in most sandwiches are minimal at best and low at worst. If you were to eat only the inside part — between the two slices — be it cheese, chicken, meat, or peanut butter, hunger would erupt within the hour. It is the bread that creates the sense of lasting fullness. Imagine cubes of bread in onion soup — and how quickly the fluid is absorbed and how swollen the cubes become, leaving no soup after a time. That is similar to what happens in the stomach. The bread mixes with gastric juices and swells and we feel full, but it is somewhat of a misconception, for we are not full of nutrients. We are full of empty calories if the bread was refined, and minimal calories if it was whole-grain. And empty calories translate into extra fat storage. Looking beyond the sandwich, there are many lunch choices that are easy, portable and satisfying, and that also raise nutrient levels high — creating the opportunity for continued high-nutrient support and a strong protein intake throughout the afternoon.

The highest-nutrient lunch you can eat is a large salad, followed with one or two fresh fruit and a high-protein food such as raw, unsalted nuts. It is really filling! Other good high-protein choices instead are a bowlful of tofu or beans, 2 to 4 ounces of goat or sheep cheese, egg salad, or fish.

Excellent nuts to eat are almonds, filberts, walnuts, pecans, pistachios, pumpkin seeds, and sunflower seeds. The white nuts — brazil nuts, whole cashews, pine nuts and macadamia nuts — are better consumed only once a week due to their higher fat content. Nut butters are also excellent, especially on celery sticks, apple slices or rice cakes. The highest-nutrient nut butters are almond butter and sesame butter, and occasionally pure peanut butter. Instead of eating nuts separately, they can be sprinkled on a salad to create a crunchy texture.

If you want to lose weight, I suggest you eat no more than 3 to 4 ounces of nuts at a meal, and do not snack on them at any other time.

A balanced lunch includes some rest time. The majority of people on the planet take siestas after lunch, resting or napping, giving the body full use of its energy to focus on digestion and renewal. In the past, for children at school, lunch was always followed by a rest period. In this hectic world, jammed with too much to do, that needed period of balance is sacrificed. Lunches have become too short and, for many, there is even no place to rest. If possible, try squeezing in a little shut-eye or quiet time and your body will thank you.

Salads

Rainbow Salad
Spinach and Arugula Salad
Coleslaw Salad with Dressing
Oriental Salad
Greek Salad
Blended Salad/Avocado Gaspachio

Rice Salad with Dressing
Cool Cucumber Salad
Mixed Bean Salad with Dressing

Dressings and Sauces

Creamy Dressing
Lemon Olive Oil Garlicky Dressing
Olive Sesame Dressing
Mustard Olive Oil Dressing
Tahini Sauce
Scrumptious Sauce
Mushroom Onion Gravy

Dips, Spreads, and Pita Pockets

Guacamole
Guacamole Veggie Pita Pocket
Hummus
Hummus Pita Pocket
Lentil Paté Dip or Spread
Falafels
Tofu Egg Salad Dip or Spread (without eggs)
Carrot Cashew Nut Paté or Spread
Bean and Veggie Tostada on Corn Tortillas

High-Nutrient Dinner Choices

Dinner is the reward at the end of the day, a time to regroup and replenish the nutrients that were used during the afternoon. It is also time to gather the rich resources for deep repair and regeneration work that intensify once we fall asleep and surrender our body to its inner intelligence. If raw materials are made up of minimal nutrients, then the body only does its basic renewal work for the next day. If raw materials are abundant and rich with nutrients, not only does the body do its renewing magic, but it has the opportunity to address any area in the body in need of attention. This can mean clearing out ingested toxins, impacted waste or clogging build-up, and repair or replacement of weak, degenerative or damaged tissue.

To best flush out any waste, as well as the residues of the deep cleansing and repair processes, it is important to have a meal containing a good amount of high-water-content foods as well as those with high nutrients. Protein intake can be minimal at night, whereas fiber to move waste out of the body, complex carbohydrates, starches, and a rich array of vitamins, minerals, and essential fats will fuel and empower any nighttime work that is needed.

Starting dinner with a salad guarantees a plentiful amount of basic nutrients. There are many varieties of salads to whet different appetites and appease different palates. (See salad suggestions in Lunch section above.)

Dinner Recipes

Main Courses

Spaghetti Squash with Tomato Tofu Veggie Sauce
Brown Rice and Veggies with Chopped Avocado
Vegetable Lasagna
Spaghetti (Squash) Tossed in Olive Oil and Garlic
Vegetable Burritos
Yummy Pizza Topping
with Polenta Pizza Crust
or Crispy Pizza Crust
Quick Chili
Pecan-Encrusted Fish
Baked Wild Salmon with Lemon and Dill

Tasty Steamed Veggies with one of the following potato recipes:
Baked French Fries
Mashed Potatoes
Parsley Potatoes
Baked Stuffed Potatoes

Baked Yams with Orange

Soups

Black Bean and Corn Soup
Lentil Soup with Chopped Avocado
20-Minute Miso/Vegetable/Lima Bean Soup
Cioppino (Italian Fish Stew)
Pumpkin Yam Soup
Summer Borsch
Cream of Vegetable Soup

Desserts

Desserts are best consumed as occasional treats or for special occasions, except for a piece of fruit or a bowl of popcorn, which can be snacked on daily. When eating one, it is best to wait 45 minutes to an hour after dinner; there is always a chance of complex food combining, creating digestive discomfort.

Desserts

Melon Salad with Tahini Dressing
Banana Ice Cream
Mango Strawberry Mousse
Strawberry Tofu Cheesecake
Crust for Strawberry Tofu Cheesecake
Baked Apples with Raisins and Pecans
Baked Pears with Cinnamon
Nut Date Balls
Pumpkin Pie and Pie Crust

High-Nutrient Holiday Dinner Menu

Festive Salad with Dried Cranberries

Thanksgiving Veggie Turkey Roast
with Mushroom Onion Gravy
Yam Orange Cups
Tofu Pumpkin Pie
with Banana Ice Cream

Treats

Treats are important to include in any healthy program – not only for youngsters, but also for the kid in all of us. (This is important to acknowledge and not ignore, as long as our inner child is not the one in control of our other food choices.) For children and teens, having a big bowl of popcorn on the table when getting home from school is always a good treat. And taking treats to work for those late afternoon pick-me-ups is a great way to tide one over until dinner — though offices and schools can be challenges with junk foods easily available. Having one's own healthful treats helps one squeeze by these temptations and feel satisfied at the same time.

Treats

Apple Slices with Nut Butter
Almond Bread
Olive Oil Garlic Butter
Apple Jack Bread
Roasted Garbanzo Bean Nuts
Popcorn
Corn Chips with Salsa or Guacamole
Fruit Juice Ice Pops
Hummus Dip with Carrot/Celery Sticks

Beverages

Beverages are the great American habit, from Coca Cola to

Gatorade. Popular commercial beverages contribute to obesity and diabetes almost more than any other food. Most popular beverages are basically all chemical — they are definitely "not the real thing." Even fruit smoothies, advertised as healthy alternatives, are so high in fruit sugar that weight gain is almost guaranteed. When thirsty, water is always the best for the body — adding fresh lemon or lime juice turns it into more of a treat drink. A tasty and refreshing drink is iced, non-caffeinated herbal tea, which can be kept in the fridge for days. These types of teas can be found in a huge variety of flavors, many of which are naturally sweet. When it comes to beverages, it is best to drink before a meal, not during, as the liquid will dilute the digestive enzymes in the stomach, contributing to slower digestion and sometimes even stomach aches.

Everyday low calorie beverages can include lemon flush and herbal ice tea. The rest of the beverages are higher calorie foods and are meant for special occasions- except for a little almond-banana milk used with cereals.

Beverages

Lemon Flush
Iced Herb Tea
Protein Smoothie
Natural Soda Pop
Almond Milk or Almond Banana Milk
Rice Milk

[See Chapter 6 for recipes details]

Chapter 6
The Figtree Food Program
Recipes

Y ou can still have many of the foods you love; they just
need to be prepared in a more healthful way. That is what
these recipes are all about. If there are any ingredients
you strongly dislike, leave them out or substitute something
else. Be creative and enjoy!

Organic food is preferable if available. Its nutrient base is usually stronger and it is free of toxic pesticides.

Most recipes are for single servings, unless indicated otherwise.

Breakfast Recipes

Freshly Made Juices

Breakfast Recipes

Freshly Made Juices

A juice extractor is needed to make juices. Drink them within 10 minutes of juicing, as juices oxidize quickly and lose some of their good nutrients.

Carrot Celery Juice

Ingredients

- 2 carrots, medium-size
- 2 celery stalks
- *Optional:* small chunk of ginger root, handful of parsley or cilantro, chunk of beet, 1/2 cucumber, or kale leaf

Instructions

☐ Wash and cut up ingredients. Put through juicer and sip slowly.

Mixed Veggie Juice

Ingredients

- 1 tomato
- handful of parsley or cilantro
- 1/2 cucumber
- 2 celery stalks
- *Optional:* juice of 1/2 lemon, small garlic clove to make it spicy

Instructions

☐ Wash and cut up ingredients. Put through juicer starting with tomato, then parsley or cilantro, and finish with cucumber and celery. This juice separates quickly, so be sure to stir well before sipping slowly.

Note: Encouraging kids to try a veggie juice can sometimes be difficult. For this very important introduction, making a sweeter juice can be more enticing. Try juicing 1 apple, 1 carrot, and 1 celery stalk together. Gradually over time, decrease the apple and increase the carrot and celery.

Fresh Fruit Ambrosia with Chopped Nut Topping

Ingredients

- 3 fruits, cut into bite-size pieces
- 1 tablespoon coconut flakes, dried
- 1 celery stalk, chopped finely, or 1 romaine lettuce leaf, shredded *(A green vegetable provides strong fiber so that the fruit sugar enters the bloodstream more evenly.)*
- 2 oz. walnuts, pecans or almonds, raw, unsalted, and chopped finely
- water as needed
- *Optional: 2 tablespoons tahini mixed with1 to 2 tablespoons carrot juice*

Instructions

☐ Mix together fruits and coconut flakes with chopped celery or shredded romaine lettuce leaf.

☐ Sprinkle chopped nuts on top.

☐ *Optional: Instead of nuts, try tahini thinned with carrot juice or water. Mix into fruit salad, coating all the fruit. Yum!*

Creamy Cinnamon Oatmeal Cooked with Fruit

Ingredients
- 1/2 cup natural oats (not instant)
- 1 apple, chopped, or 1/2 cup blueberries, or sliced banana, or 1/3 cup raisins, unsulphured
- 1/2 teaspoon cinnamon
- 1 1/2 cups water
- *Optional:* 1/4 cup walnuts, raw and chopped (for extra protein) Almond Banana Milk or soy milk, unsweetened

Instructions
- ☐ Boil water
- ☐ Add oats, apple or other fruit, plus cinnamon (and chopped nuts).
- ☐ Cover and simmer (about 8 to 10 minutes), stirring every few minutes.
- ☐ The oatmeal should be creamy and not need any other liquid, but Almond Banana Milk (recipe on page 94), or unsweetened soy milk may be added if desired.

Veggie Avocado Omelet with Salsa

Ingredients
- 2 large eggs, beaten
- 1/2 small onion, chopped
- 1 roma tomato, chopped
- 1/2 red bell pepper, chopped
- 1 small zucchini, chopped
- small handful of spinach, or chard leaf, chopped
- 1 tablespoon olive oil
- 1/2 avocado, sliced
- Salsa (recipe on page 90)

Instructions
- ☐ Steam all the chopped veggies for 5 minutes.
- ☐ In a cast-iron frying pan heat 1 tablespoon of olive oil, then add eggs to cover entire bottom of pan.
- ☐ Add cooked veggies on one half, cover with lid and cook another 5 minutes or until the egg has solidified.
- ☐ Fold over and serve with avocado slices and salsa on top.

Note: Originally I made this recipe in a Teflon-coated pan without using oil. But recent information has surfaced about the long-term toxic effects of using Teflon, and now I prefer cast iron. Ask anyone with a pet bird about Teflon — they will tell you that if the heat gets high enough on Teflon, the fumes can actually kill their bird. .

Breakfast Lunch Dinner Dessert Treats Beverages

Banana Walnut Pancakes

Ingredients
- 2 large eggs, beaten
- 1 banana, ripe (brown spots on skin) and mashed, or 1 apple, grated
- 1/2 teaspoon cinnamon
- 1/4 cup walnuts, chopped
- olive oil as needed

Instructions
- ☐ Mix above ingredients together.
- ☐ In a cast-iron frying pan heat a thin layer of olive oil to coat bottom.
- ☐ When the oil is hot, pour mixture into pan with a ladle forming 2- to 3-inch pancakes.
- ☐ When little bubbles begin to form on top of pancake, flip over and brown other side.
- ☐ Serve immediately.

This recipe is my favorite treat. It is also delicious when a grated apple is substituted for the banana.

Muesli with Fresh Fruit, Seeds, and Banana Almond Milk

Ingredients

- 1/3 cup oat flakes
- 1/3 cup barley flakes
- 1/3 cup rye flakes
- 1/4 cup sunflower seeds
- 1/8 cup raisins, unsulphured
- 1/8 cup coconut, dried and shredded (no additives)
- olive oil as needed
- 1 apple, chopped, or 4 strawberries or other fruit, chopped Almond Milk or Banana Almond Milk

Instructions

- ☐ Preheat oven to 250°F.
- ☐ Mix together all dried ingredients. With olive oil, grease cookie sheet and spread dried mixture evenly over surface. Bake for 10 minutes.
- ☐ Add remaining ingredients.
- ☐ Pour Almond Milk or Banana Almond Milk (recipes on page 90) over cereal and enjoy!

Note: Larger quantities can be made and stored. Or for more instant muesli, blend all flakes in blender, then pour into bowl.

Breakfast Lunch Dinner Dessert Treats Beverages

Millet Waffles

Ingredients

- 2 cups millet
- 2 tablespoons olive oil
- 2 tablespoons pure maple syrup
- 1/2 teaspoon salt
- 1/2 teaspoon coriander, ground
- 2 1/2 cups water
- cinnamon to taste
- 4 strawberries, sliced

Instructions

☐ Wash millet and put in large bowl with 1 1/2 cups water and soak overnight.

☐ Drain and rinse millet and put in blender with 1 cup water and the remaining ingredients.

☐ Blend to a thick batter.

☐ Pour some batter onto a hot waffle iron, close and bake.

☐ Repeat with remaining batter.

☐ Dust with cinnamon and serve with strawberries on top.

Scrambled Tofu

(Serves 4)

Ingredients

- 1 lb. tofu, organic and firm
- 1 tablespoon tamari sauce
- 1 teaspoon curry powder or turmeric
- 1/2 onion, diced
- 1 red bell pepper, diced
- handful of mushrooms, sliced (preferably shiitake)
- 1 zucchini, diced olive oil as needed
- *Optional: black pepper to taste*

Instructions

- ☐ Take tofu out of water and mush it into a bowl.
- ☐ Add tamari sauce and curry powder.
- ☐ Mix well and set aside.
- ☐ Steam onion, red bell pepper, mushrooms and zucchini.
- ☐ Spice up with black pepper if desired.
- ☐ Heat a little olive oil in frying pan.
- ☐ Add tofu and steamed veggies and stir well. Sauté for 5 minutes and serve.

Contributed by Beatrix Rohlsen from *The Art of Taste*

Lunch Recipes

Salads

Dressings and Sauces

Dips, Spreads, and Pita Pockets

Rainbow Salad

Ingredients

- 3 to 4 leaves of romaine or other red or green lettuce (except iceberg)
- 6 cherry tomatoes, sliced in half, or 1 tomato, chopped
- 1/2 red bell pepper, sweet and chopped
- 1/2 cucumber, (peeled, if waxed), chopped
- 1 carrot, grated
- 1 celery stalk, chopped
- small chunk of red onion, chopped
- 4 kalamata olives, pitted and chopped
- *Optional:* handful of sunflower sprouts, chopped, or any additional raw vegetables of your choice

Instructions

☐ Cut up ingredients and mix in bowl. Pour dressing of your choice over and toss.

Spinach and Arugula Salad

Ingredients

- 2 cups baby spinach leaves, coarsely chopped
- 1 cup arugula leaves, coarsely chopped
- handful of cherry tomatoes, sliced in half
- 1/2 red onion, chopped
- 1/2 red bell pepper, chopped
- handful of kalamata black olives, pitted and chopped
- *Optional: 2 oz. crumbled sheep or goat feta cheese*

Instructions

☐ Mix all ingredients together and sprinkle with Lemon/Olive Oil Dressing (recipe on page 50).

Greek Salad

Ingredients

- 2 ripe tomatoes, coarsely chopped
- 1/2 red bell pepper, coarsely chopped
- 1 cucumber, coarsely chopped
- 1/2 red onion, chopped
- 8 black kalamata olives, pitted and chopped
- 1/4 lb. crumbled goat or sheep feta cheese
- sprinkle of olive oil
- 1/2 lemon, juiced

Instructions

☐ Mix together all salad ingredients. Sprinkle with olive oil and lemon juice.

Blended Salad/Avocado Gaspachio

Ingredients

- 1 tomato
- 1/2 red bell pepper
- 1/2 cucumber
- 1/4 red onion
- small handful of cilantro
- 1/2 avocado
- 1/2 lemon, juiced
- 4 leaves romaine lettuce
- 1 celery stalk

Instructions

☐ Cut up all ingredients (except celery stalk) and blend in food processor or blender (in blender push down mixture with celery stalk)

☐ Serve immediately.

Breakfast **Lunch** Dinner Dessert Treats Beverages

Breakfast **Lunch** Dinner Dessert Treats Beverages

Coleslaw Salad

Ingredients
- 4 cups white cabbage, shredded
- 2 celery stalks, finely chopped
- 1 small sweet apple, finely chopped
- 1 large carrot, grated
- 2 tablespoons walnuts, coarsely chopped

Instructions
☐ Mix together all ingredients in a large bowl and serve with Mustard/Olive Oil Dressing (below).

Mustard/Olive Oil Dressing

Ingredients
- 3 tablespoons olive oil
- 1 spring onion, finely chopped
- 1/2 teaspoon mustard
- 1 tablespoon lemon juice

Instructions
☐ In a jar mix together all dressing ingredients, shake, pour over Coleslaw Salad (above), and toss.

Oriental Salad

Ingredients
- 1/2 cabbage, shredded
- 1/2 cup carrot, grated
- 2 celery stalks, chopped
- 1/2 red onion, chopped
- 1 cup bean sprouts

Instructions
☐ Mix together ingredients and sprinkle with Olive Sesame Dressing (recipe on page 51)

Breakfast **Lunch** Dinner Dessert Treats Beverages

Breakfast **Lunch** Dinner Dessert Treats Beverages

Mixed Bean Salad

(Serves 6)

Ingredients
- 4 cups beans, cooked (1 1/3 cup of each: kidney, black, Anasazi)
- 2 large red onions, diced
- 2 large tomatoes, diced
- 1/2 cup cilantro, chopped
- 4 cobs corn, cooked separately and cut off the cob

Instructions
- ☐ In a large bowl mix all ingredients together.
- ☐ Toss with dressing.

Dressing for Mixed Bean Salad

Ingredients
- 4 tablespoons olive oil
- 2 tablespoons balsamic vinegar
- 2 garlic cloves, crushed
- salt and pepper to taste

Instructions
- ☐ Mix all ingredients together in bowl.
- ☐ Toss with salad.

Contributed by Nadia Natali, from *Cooking Off the Grid*

Rice Salad

(Serves 6)

Ingredients
- 2 cups brown rice, cooked
- 1 cucumber, cubed
- 1 tomato, fresh, cubed
- 1 red pepper, diced
- 1 green pepper, diced
- 1 red onion, diced
- 1/4 cup cilantro or parsley
- 1/4 teaspoon salt

Instructions
- ☐ In a large bowl mix all ingredients together.
- ☐ Toss with dressing.

Dressing for Rice Salad

Ingredients
- 2 tablespoons rice vinegar
- 4 tablespoons apple juice
- 1 tablespoon tamari soy sauce
- 1 tablespoon olive oil

Instructions
- ☐ Mix all ingredients together in bowl.
- ☐ Toss with salad

Contributed by Nadia Natali, from *Cooking Off the Grid*

Breakfast **Lunch** Dinner Dessert Treats Beverages

Cool Cucumber Salad

(Serves 6)

Ingredients

- 1 large cucumber, sliced very thin
- 1/2 red onion, sliced very thin
- 2 tablespoons rice vinegar
- 1 tablespoon lime or lemon, juiced
- 1/8 teaspoon salt

Instructions

☐ In a medium shallow bowl place all the ingredients and toss.

☐ Sprinkle with 1 teaspoon dill, dried or chopped.

Contributed by Nadia Natali, from *Cooking Off the Grid*

Mustard Olive Oil Dressing

Ingredients

- 3 tablespoons olive oil
- 1 spring onion, finely chopped
- 1/2 teaspoon mustard
- 1 tablespoon lemon juice

Instructions

☐ Blend all ingredients in a blender or shake in a tightly closed jar. Can be stored in a dark cabinet.

Scrumptious Sauce

(Makes 5 cups)

Ingredients
- 4 cups olive oil
- 1/2 cup Braggs Liquid Aminos
- 1/2 cup yeast flakes
- 1/2 teaspoon kelp powder
- 1/2 teaspoon basil
- 2 garlic cloves, crushed
- 1 1/2 teaspoon lemon juice

Instructions
- ☐ Blend all ingredients in blender for 1 minute.
- ☐ Store in a cabinet. Do not refrigerate.

Notes: Excellent on salads, vegetables, grains and potatoes

Tahini Sauce

Ingredients
- 1 cup tahini (sesame butter)
- 1/8 cup lemon juice
- 1 garlic clove, crushed
- 1 tablespoon tamari sauce
- water to thin

Instructions
- ☐ Squeeze lemon juice into tahini, add tamari sauce and garlic clove and mix.
- ☐ Slowly add a little water until consistency of tahini becomes more liquid and pourable but not thin.

Breakfast Lunch Dinner Dessert Treats Beverages

Creamy Dressing

Ingredients

- 1 cup olive oil
- 1/2 lemon, juiced
- 1 tablespoon balsamic vinegar
- 1 tablespoon tamari or soy sauce
- 1 tablespoon brewer's yeast flakes
- 1 garlic clove, crushed
- 1/3 cup water

Instructions

☐ Blend all ingredients in blender.

☐ Pour into jar to save.

☐ Use 1 or 2 tablespoons per salad.

☐ Do not refrigerate, but keep in a dark cool place.

Lemon Olive Oil Garlicky Dressing

Ingredients

- 1 cup olive oil
- 1 lemon, juiced
- 1 garlic clove, crushed
- 1/2 cup water
- *Optional: 1 teaspoon white miso paste, shake of black pepper, dried mustard, oregano, and dill or basil*

Instructions

☐ Blend all ingredients in blender.

☐ Pour into jar to save.

☐ Use 1 or 2 tablespoons per salad.

☐ Do not refrigerate, but keep in a dark cool place.

Olive Sesame Dressing

Ingredients
- 1/2 cup olive oil
- 1 teaspoon sesame seed oil, toasted
- 1 tablespoon balsamic vinegar
- 1 tablespoon tamari sauce
- 1/2 cup water

Instructions
- ☐ Blend all ingredients in a blender or shake in a tightly closed jar. Can be stored in a dark cabinet.

Mushroom Onion Gravy

Ingredients
- 1 medium onion, chopped
- 2 tablespoons olive oil
- 2 1/2 cups water
- 2 tablespoons cornstarch
- 1 tablespoon tamari sauce
- 1/2 teaspoon rosemary, dried
- 1/2 teaspoon thyme, dried
- 1/4 teaspoon sage, dried
- 1 teaspoon miso paste
- 1 bay leaf
- 4 oz. mushrooms, sliced (shiitake are best)

Instructions
- ☐ Sauté onion in saucepan with olive oil for 5 minutes.
- ☐ Mix cornstarch with 4 tablespoon of water, making a smooth white liquid.
- ☐ Slowly add cornstarch mixture to pan of onions, stirring continuously until absorbed.
- ☐ Mix in remaining ingredients.
- ☐ Cover partially with lid and continue to stir occasionally until sauce thickens (about 20 minutes).

Breakfast **Lunch** Dinner Dessert Treats Beverages

Guacamole

Ingredients
- 1 avocado, mashed with lemon juice
- 1/2 onion, chopped
- 1/2 lemon, juiced
- 1 teaspoon tamari sauce

Instructions
☐ Mix onion, lemon juice, and tamari sauce with mashed avocado.

Veggie Pita Pocket

Ingredients
- 1 romaine lettuce leaf, shredded
- 1 tomato, chopped
- 1/2 carrot, grated
- a handful sunflower sprouts, chopped
- 2 tablespoons sunflower seeds, raw
- 2 tablespoons tahini sauce
- 1 whole wheat pita pocket

Instructions
☐ To the guacamole mixture, add shredded romaine lettuce, chopped tomato, grated carrot, sunflower sprouts and seeds.

☐ Mix in 2 tablespoons Tahini Sauce (recipe on page 49).

☐ Place mixture inside two halves of a whole wheat pita pocket.

Note: Dips, Spreads, and Pita Pockets can also be served with raw veggie sticks, almond bread, or in corn tortillas.

Hummus

Ingredients
- 1 cup chickpeas, cooked
- 1/4 cup water
- 1/2 lemon, juiced
- dash of paprika
- 1 teaspoon tamari sauce
- 1 garlic clove

Instructions
- ☐ Put chickpeas in blender with other ingredients and blend until smooth.

Hummus Pita Pocket

Ingredients
- 1 cup hummus
- 1 romaine lettuce leaf, shredded
- 1 tomato, sliced
- 1 carrot, grated
- handful of sunflower
- sprouts, chopped
- 1 whole grain pita pocket

- *Optional: 1 tablespoon tahini sauce*

Instructions
- ☐ Stuff pita pocket with hummus and other ingredients. For extra creaminess, add tahini sauce.

Breakfast **Lunch** *Dinner Dessert Treats Beverages*

Breakfast Lunch Dinner Dessert Treats Beverages

Lentil Paté Dip or Spread

Ingredients

- 1/2 cup red lentils
- 1/2 onion, medium-size and chopped
- 1 carrot, medium-size and grated
- 1 garlic clove, crushed
- 1 teaspoon cumin, ground
- 1/2 teaspoon turmeric
- 2 tablespoons tamari sauce
- 1/2 cup cilantro, finely chopped
- 1 1/2 cups water
- 2 teaspoons olive oil

Instructions

- ☐ Place lentils and water in saucepan and bring to boil. Then cover and simmer for 40 minutes.
- ☐ In a cast-iron frying pan heat olive oil, then reduce heat and add onion, carrot and garlic. Sauté and stir until carrots are soft.
- ☐ Remove from heat and add in remaining ingredients.
- ☐ Add in red lentils after they are cooked.
- ☐ Allow paté to cool before serving.

Carrot Cashew Nut Paté or Spread

Ingredients

- 1 1/2 cups carrots, sliced
- 1 cup cashews, whole (cashew pieces tend to be rancid)
- 1/2 teaspoon orange rind, grated
- 1 tablespoon spring onions, chopped
- black pepper to taste
- 1 tablespoon orange juice
- 1 teaspoon tamari sauce

Instructions

- ☐ Steam carrots until just soft.
- ☐ Blend cashews in a food processor or blender until finely ground.
- ☐ Add the remaining ingredients and blend until smooth.
- ☐ If dry, add a little more orange juice.

Tofu Egg Salad Dip or Spread (without eggs)

Ingredients
- 1 lb. tofu, firm
- 2 tablespoons mustard
- 1 tablespoon tamari sauce
- 1/2 teaspoon turmeric
- 4 scallions, finely chopped
- 1 celery stalk, finely chopped

Instructions
- ☐ Drain tofu and mash in a bowl. Add all other ingredients, mixing well.
- ☐ Chill at least 1 hour before serving.

Falafels

Ingredients
- 1 potato, baked or steamed
- 2 cups garbanzo beans, cooked
- 3 tablespoons tahini
- 1/2 cup parsley, minced
- 1/2 onion, finely chopped
- 2 garlic cloves, crushed
- 1 tablespoon tamari sauce
- 1 teaspoon paprika
- olive oil as needed
- 1 leaf romaine lettuce, chopped
- 1/2 tomato, chopped

Instructions
- ☐ Mash cooked potato, then puree garbanzo beans in blender.
- ☐ Add all ingredients in a bowl and mix together.
- ☐ Drop by spoonfuls on an olive oil–greased baking pan and bake for 25 minutes at 350°F.
- ☐ Can be served on top of a salad or stuffed inside whole wheat pita bread with chopped lettuce and tomato, and Tahini Sauce (recipe on page 49).

Bean and Veggie Tostada on Corn Tortillas

Ingredients

- 2 cups black or pinto beans (soaked overnight and cooked in fresh water until soft, or canned without preservatives)
- 1/2 onion, chopped
- 1 tomato, chopped
- 1/2 red bell pepper, chopped
- 1 celery stalk, chopped
- 1 carrot, grated
- handful of cilantro, chopped

- 2 corn tortillas
- 2 leaves romaine lettuce, shredded
- 1/2 avocado, chopped
- *Optional: tofu mozzarella cheese, grated*

Instructions

☐ In a cooking pan add beans, onion, tomato, bell pepper, celery, and cilantro and heat slowly, stirring frequently until hot but not boiling.

☐ Warm tortillas over flame on top of stove or heat in 250°F oven for 5 minutes.

☐ Place bean mixture on tortillas, top with shredded romaine lettuce, grated carrot, and chopped avocado.

☐ Grated tofu mozzarella cheese can be sprinkled on top of the dish and placed for 1 minute under a broiler or in toaster oven.

Dinner Recipes

Main Courses

Soups

Holiday Dinner Menu

Breakfast Lunch **Dinner** Dessert Treats Beverages

Vegetable Lasagna

Ingredients

- 2 cups tomato puree
- 1/2 teaspoon oregano
- 2 garlic cloves, crushed
- 4 large potatoes, sliced
- 1/4 inch thick
- 1 large eggplant, sliced
- 1/4 inch thick
- 1 large onion, sliced
- 2 cups chard, chopped
- 2 zucchini, sliced
- 1/4 inch thick
- 1 cup mushrooms, sliced
- olive oil as needed
- 1/2 cup water
- 1 cup tofu mozzarella cheese, grated

Instructions

- ☐ Oil an 8-inch casserole dish and grease bottom and sides with olive oil.
- ☐ To the tomato puree, mix in oregano and garlic. Spread 2 tablespoons of tomato puree mixture on bottom, then place one layer of potato slices over that.
- ☐ Continue, adding 1 tablespoon of tomato puree between each layer.
- ☐ The next layer, add eggplant slices. Repeat another layer of potatoes followed with another layer of eggplant. The next layer, add onion slices, and then a layer of chard, and then a layer of mushrooms. Add a layer of eggplant next, and finish with a top layer of zucchini.
- ☐ Add remaining tomato puree on top. Sprinkle with 1/2 cup water and bake in a 400°F oven for 1 hour.
- ☐ Five minutes before it's finished, sprinkle on top grated tofu mozzarella cheese.

Note: To get the highest nutrient intake, be sure to start with a salad. Most of these recipes make 4 servings.

Spaghetti Squash with Tomato Tofu Veggie Sauce

Ingredients
- 1 large spaghetti squash

Instructions
- ☐ Preheat oven to 350°F. Make several fork holes in squash and bake for 1 hour.

Sauce Ingredients
- 2 cups tomatoes, fresh and chopped, or one 16 oz. can tomatoes, chopped
- 1 eggplant, chopped into
- 1/2 inch cubes
- 1 zucchini, chopped
- 4 to 6 shiitake mushrooms, coarsely chopped
- 1 onion, chopped
- 1 carrot, finely chopped
- 2 garlic cloves, crushed
- 1 teaspoon oregano
- 2 cups water
- 2 tablespoons tamari sauce
- 1 tablespoon olive oil
- *Optional: 1 cup tofu, soft and crumbled*

Sauce Instructions
- ☐ Place ingredients except olive oil and tamari sauce in a pot with 1 1/2 inches of water. Bring to boil, then cover and simmer 35 minutes.
- ☐ When finished, add olive oil and tamari sauce.
- ☐ This recipe also can be blended when finished, creating a smooth tomato sauce. (Blended tomato sauce is great for kids who don't like the sight of vegetables!)
- ☐ When spaghetti squash is cooked, cut through the middle, not lengthwise.
- ☐ Scoop out and discard seeds. With fork, pull out spaghetti-like strands and place on platter.
- ☐ Pour sauce on top and toss.

Brown Rice and Veggies with Chopped Avocado

Ingredients
- 2 cups brown rice
- 2 zucchini, chopped
- 1 large carrot, chopped
- 4 chard leaves, chopped
- 1 white onion, chopped
- 1 cup corn kernels
- 1 cup string beans, chopped
- 6 cups water
- 1 avocado, chopped

Instructions
- ☐ Bring water to boil, add brown rice and all other ingredients, cover and simmer for 45 minutes or until all water is absorbed.
- ☐ Serve with chopped avocado garnish.

Spaghetti (Squash) Tossed in Olive Oil and Garlic

Ingredients
- 1 spaghetti squash, medium-size 4 tablespoons olive oil
- 3 garlic cloves, crushed
- 1/8 teaspoon black pepper
- 2 tablespoons tamari sauce

Instructions
- ☐ Wash spaghetti squash and pierce five times with a fork.
- ☐ Bake in 375°F oven for 1 hour.
- ☐ Halve squash through the middle and clean out seeds.
- ☐ With a fork, pull out long strands of squash.
- ☐ Heat olive oil, then add garlic and cook about 2 minutes until garlic begins to slightly crisp.
- ☐ Remove from heat, add pepper and tamari sauce, and toss with squash until thoroughly coated.

Vegetable Burritos

Sauce Ingredients

- 1 onion, chopped
- 2 garlic cloves, crushed
- 1/3 cup green chilies, canned and chopped
- 1 tablespoon chili powder
- 1 teaspoon cumin, ground
- 1/8 teaspoon cayenne
- 6 oz. can tomato paste
- 1 cup tomatoes, chopped
- 1 tablespoon olive oil

Sauce Instructions

- ☐ Place all ingredients in saucepan.
- ☐ Heat until it boils. Then cover and simmer for 30 minutes.

Filling Ingredients

- 1 onion, chopped
- 1 green bell pepper, chopped
- 1 cup corn kernels
- 2 cups zucchini, chopped
- 1 cup mushrooms, chopped
- 1/2 teaspoon chili powder
- 1 teaspoon cumin, ground
- 8 corn flour tortillas
- 2 tablespoons olive oil
- 1/3 cup water

Filling Instructions

- ☐ Sauté all ingredients in olive oil for 2 minutes.
- ☐ Add water, cover and simmer for another 10 minutes.
- ☐ Place 1/3 cup of filling down the center of a tortilla.
- ☐ Pour 2 tablespoons sauce on top of filling.
- ☐ Roll up tortillas and enjoy.

Breakfast Lunch **Dinner** Dessert Treats Beverages

Breakfast   Lunch   **Dinner**   Dessert   Treats   Beverages

Yummy Pizza Sauce

Ingredients

- 1/2 teaspoon oregano, dried
- 1 cup tomato, pureed
- 1/2 small onion, chopped
- 1 cup shiitake mushrooms, sliced
- 10 kalamata olives, pitted and chopped

Instructions

- ☐ Place all ingredients in saucepan, bring to boil, then cover and simmer for 5 minutes.
- ☐ Spread pizza sauce on top of crust. You can choose a crust from one of the two pizza crust recipes that follow (recipes on pages 62 or 63). They are both delicious.

Polenta Pizza Crust

Ingredients

- 2/3 cup polenta flour
- 2 2/3 cups water
- 1 tablespoon olive oil
- 1 cup tofu mozzarella cheese, grated

Instructions

- ☐ Mix polenta flour with 2/3 cup cold water in a pan.
- ☐ Add 2 cups of boiling water, mixing constantly.
- ☐ Bring to a boil and simmer over low heat, continuing to stir for 5 minutes.
- ☐ Beat in the olive oil. Grease a 10- to 12-inch pizza pan and spread polenta mixture to form pizza.
- ☐ Spread sauce on top.
- ☐ Bake in oven at 400°F for 30 minutes.
- ☐ Sprinkle with tofu mozzarella cheese and cook for 3 more minutes.

Crispy Pizza Crust

Ingredients
- 1 large egg
- 1 teaspoon olive oil
- 1 cup almond flour
- 1/4 teaspoon kosher salt

Instructions
- ☐ In a bowl with a wooden spoon, mix all the ingredients well and form a ball.
- ☐ Using a parchment-covered baking sheet or an oiled pizza pan, press the dough into a round pizza shape, using your hands.
- ☐ Put the pizza in a cold oven and heat to 300°F. Cook until pizza gets golden brown and crispy, about 30 minutes.
- ☐ Top with Yummy Pizza Sauce (recipe on page 62) and bake for 20 minutes more.

Contributed by Kendall Conrad, from *Eat Well, Feel Well*

Quick Chili

Ingredients
- 1/2 cup water
- 2 onions, chopped
- 1 green pepper, chopped
- 1 celery stalk, chopped
- 1 garlic clove, crushed
- 4 cups tomatoes, fresh or canned
- 4 cups kidney beans, cooked
- 2 tablespoons chili powder
- 2 teaspoons cumin, ground
- olive oil as needed

Instructions
- ☐ Sauté onions, green pepper, celery and garlic in a small amount of olive oil for 5 minutes.
- ☐ Add remaining ingredients, cover and simmer for another 25 minutes.
- ☐ Stir occasionally. Can be served over brown rice or baked potato.

Pecan-Encrusted Fish

Ingredients
- 1 1/2 lbs. unfarmed white fish (mahi mahi, halibut, sea bass or others)
- 1 cup pecans, raw
- 1/2 cup lemon juice
- 2 tablespoons tamari sauce
- 2 garlic cloves, crushed
- olive oil as needed

Instructions
- ☐ Preheat oven to 350°F.
- ☐ In blender, blend pecans into small pieces. Place on a flat plate.
- ☐ Mix together lemon juice, tamari sauce, and crushed garlic and pour over both sides of fish. Then press fish into pecan mixture, one side and then the next.
- ☐ Press remaining pecan pieces on top of fish.
- ☐ Place in olive-oiled glass baking dish and bake for 15 to 20 minutes.

Baked Wild Salmon with Lemon and Dill

Ingredients
- 1 1/2 lbs. wild salmon
- 1 lemon small bunch fresh dill,
- chopped black pepper to taste
- 2 garlic cloves, crushed
- olive oil as needed

Instructions
- ☐ Preheat oven to 350°F.
- ☐ Place fish in olive-oiled baking pan.
- ☐ Squeeze lemon over fish.
- ☐ Sprinkle over with black pepper and chopped dill.
- ☐ Cover and bake for 15 to 20 minutes.

Tasty Steamed Veggies

Ingredients

Select a variety of vegetables from the following:

- Leafy greens: chard, spinach, collard greens, mustard greens (about 5 minutes to steam, become limp when ready);
- Broccoli, cauliflower, brussel sprouts, string beans, bok choy, cabbage, peas, snow peas, corn, eggplant, onions, kale (about 8 to 10 minutes to steam);
- Beets, rutabagas, parsnips, carrots, leeks, turnips (about 12 to 15 minutes to steam) 1/2 lemon, juiced

Instructions

☐ Choose up to 1 lb. of mixed vegetables per person.

Different colors ensure a good variety of nutrients and an attractive color combination. It is best to steam vegetables as whole as possible, as this preserves the most vitamins.

☐ After steaming, they can be cut into smaller pieces.

☐ After the vegetables have been arranged on a platter, sprinkle with olive oil and lemon juice.

The olive oil enhances flavor by dissolving flavor molecules in the food, making them more available to the taste. Lemon juice brings out a natural, salty flavor in foods.

Note: *For a complete meal, serve with one of the potato recipes that follow, or a yam dish or a whole grain.*

Breakfast Lunch Dinner Dessert Treats Beverages

Baked Yams with Orange

Ingredients
- 1 lb. yams per person
- 1/2 orange per person

Instructions
- ☐ Make fork marks in yams and bake 1 hour in a 350°F oven.
- ☐ Place a sheet of aluminum foil in bottom of oven to catch drippings.
- ☐ When cooked, slice open top of yams and squeeze in juice of 1/2 orange.

Baked French Fries

Ingredients
- 1 lb. potatoes per person, sliced
- 1/4-inch thick natural mustard to taste
- ketchup, sugar-free

Instructions
- ☐ Preheat oven to 475°F.
- ☐ Place potatoes slices on oven rack for 20 minutes or until potatoes are slightly brown and puffy.
- ☐ Eat immediately. Serve with natural mustard or sugar-free ketchup.

Parsley Potatoes

Ingredients
- 4 large potatoes, cut in quarters
- 1 cup parsley, chopped
- black pepper to taste
- sprinkle of olive oil

Instructions
- ☐ Steam potatoes until soft.
- ☐ Cut into smaller chunks.
- ☐ Sprinkle parsley and black pepper over potatoes.
- ☐ Sprinkle with olive oil and toss.

Baked Stuffed Potatoes

Ingredients
- 4 large russet or yukon gold potatoes
- 1 small onion, chopped
- 2 large tomatoes, chopped
- 8 kalamata olives, pitted and chopped
- 1 tablespoon olive oil
- 1 avocado

Instructions
- ☐ Wash potatoes and bake for 1 1/4 hours in oven at 350°F.
- ☐ Sauté onion, tomatoes, and olives together for 5 minutes in olive oil.
- ☐ When finished, split potatoes in half.
- ☐ Scoop out contents and place in bowl with onion/tomato/olive mixture.
- ☐ Mash with avocado.
- ☐ Fill potatoes with warm mixture and serve immediately.

Breakfast Lunch Dinner Dessert Treats Beverages

Mashed Potatoes

Ingredients

- 6 potatoes, medium-size, peeled and cut into large chunks
- 1 onion, chopped
- 2 garlic cloves, crushed
- water as needed
- 1 tablespoon olive oil
- *Optional: 4 tablespoons parsley, chopped*

Instructions

- ☐ Place all ingredients in saucepan (except olive oil) and cover with 1 inch of water.
- ☐ Bring to a boil, cover and simmer for 20 minutes.
- ☐ Remove from heat and pour with liquid into blender.
- ☐ Add olive oil and blend until smooth.
- ☐ Serve with Mushroom Onion Gravy (recipe on page 51).

Lentil Soup with Chopped Avocado

Ingredients

- 1/2 cup red or green lentils (red lentils cook faster)
- 1 small onion, chopped
- 2 chard leaves, chopped
- 1 carrot, chopped
- 1 zucchini, chopped
- 1/2 cup corn, cut off cob or frozen

- handful of fresh dill, chopped, or 1/2 teaspoon dill, dried
- 1 tablespoon white miso
- 1 lemon, juiced
- 1 tablespoon olive oil
- 4 cups water
- 1/4 to 1/2 avocado, chopped

Instructions

- ☐ Bring water to boil, add lentils and all other vegetables including dill, cover and simmer for 30 minutes (for red lentils), or 45 minutes (for green lentils).
- ☐ Check after 15 minutes to make sure there is enough water.
- ☐ After lentils are soft, remove 1 cup soup stock and add to it white miso. Stir until dissolved.
- ☐ Add back into soup, along with olive oil and lemon juice.
- ☐ Serve chopped avocado on top as a garnish.

Note: White or yellow miso paste makes wonderful bouillon for any soup or stew — it not only adds saltiness, but has a delicious full flavor. It can be purchased in most health food stores or Oriental food markets. Miso should never be boiled, so only add it after the soup is cooked. To use it, when soup is finished and still hot, remove a cup of liquid. Depending on the amount of soup, add 1 or 2 tablespoons of miso to the cup of liquid and mash until it becomes completely dissolved. Pour back into soup and mix in.

Breakfast Lunch **Dinner** Dessert Treats Beverages

20-Minute Miso/Vegetable/Lima Bean Soup

Ingredients
- 2 bags lima beans, frozen
- 2 carrots, chopped
- 1 onion, chopped
- 2 zucchini, chopped
- bunch of fresh dill, chopped
- 1 cup corn kernels
- 2 tablespoons white or yellow miso
- water as needed
- 1 tablespoon olive oil

Instructions
- ☐ Rinse lima beans and put in pot with chopped vegetables, including dill.
- ☐ Cover with water to top of mixture. Bring to boil, cover and simmer.
- ☐ After 20 minutes turn off heat and remove 1 cup of hot liquid.
- ☐ Add miso paste to it and mix until dissolved.
- ☐ Add mixture back to soup, along with olive oil.

Cioppino (Italian Fish Stew)

Ingredients

- 1 1/2 lbs. unfarmed white fish (mahi mahi, halibut, sea bass or others)
- 4 roma tomatoes, or 8 oz. can tomatoes, chopped
- 12 kalamata olives, pitted and chopped
- 1 bunch fresh dill
- 1 onion, small and chopped
- 1 zucchini, chopped
- 20 string beans, chopped
- 3 chard leaves, chopped
- black pepper to taste
- 1 1/2 cups water
- 2 tablespoons olive oil
- tamari sauce to taste

Instructions

- ☐ Place fish, all vegetables, black pepper, and water in large pot, bring to boil, then cover and simmer for 20 minutes.
- ☐ Add olive oil, and tamari to taste.

Breakfast   Lunch   **Dinner**   Dessert   Treats   Beverages

Pumpkin Yam Soup

Ingredients

- 2 tablespoons olive oil
- 1 teaspoon fresh ginger, minced
- 1 garlic clove, minced
- 1 onion, diced
- 3 cups pumpkin, coarsely diced
- 3 cups yams, coarsely diced
- dash each of cumin, nutmeg, cayenne pepper
- 4 cups water or vegetable broth
- 1 tablespoon tamari sauce
- 1/4 bunch tarragon

Instructions

- ☐ Sauté ginger, garlic and onion in olive oil.
- ☐ Add pumpkin, yams, spices, tamari sauce, and water or vegetable broth.
- ☐ Simmer covered for 3 minutes.
- ☐ Use electric hand blender or put in blender to puree soup.
- ☐ Add tarragon and let sit for 5 minutes before serving.

Contributed by Beatrix Rohlsen from *The Art of Taste*

Summer Borsch

Ingredients
- 6 cups water
- 4 large beets, cut into large bite-size pieces, include greens
- 3 large carrots, sliced
- 2 large onions, cut into large bite-size pieces
- 8 large new potatoes, cut into large bite-size pieces

Instructions
- ☐ Steam all ingredients in a very large pot until soft.
- ☐ Add to pot in the order given while cutting. Beets take the longest to cook.
- ☐ Save broth for soup.
- ☐ Blend the vegetables in a blender with the broth. You may need to do this in two batches if your blender is small.
- ☐ If you find the proportion too dry for blending, add 1/2 cup extra liquid, such as soup broth or water. The consistency should be thick and a little rough.

Contributed by Nadia Natali, from *Cooking Off the Grid*

Cream of Vegetable Soup

Ingredients

- 1 large onion
- 1 leek
- 2 carrots
- 2 zucchini
- 3 chard leaves
- 2 medium potatoes
- water as needed
- 3 tablespoons olive oil
- 2 tablespoons white miso
- 1/2 cup fresh dill, chopped,

or 1/4 teaspoon dill, dried
- 1 avocado, chopped

Instructions

- ☐ Chop vegetables and potatoes into small chunks.
- ☐ Put in saucepan and add water to almost cover vegetables, leaving 1/2 inch of vegetables above water line.
- ☐ Bring to a boil, then cover and simmer 1/2 hour.
- ☐ When finished, place in blender with olive oil and miso and blend and serve.
- ☐ Sprinkle dill in center of each bowl of soup.
- ☐ Garnish with chopped avocado.

Breakfast Lunch Dinner Dessert Treats Beverages

Black Bean and Corn Soup

Ingredients
- 2 cups black beans, soaked overnight in water
- 2 carrots, chopped
- 1 onion, chopped
- 2 zucchini, chopped
- bunch of fresh dill, chopped
- 2 cups corn kernels
- 8 cups water
- 1 tablespoon olive oil
- tamari sauce or sea salt to taste

Instructions
- ☐ Rinse beans, put in pot with water, bring to boil, cover and simmer.
- ☐ Check after 1 hour.
- ☐ When beans are slightly soft, add remaining ingredients and continue simmering until beans are tender.
- ☐ Add olive oil, and tamari sauce or sea salt to taste.

Festive Salad with Dried Cranberries

Ingredients

- 1 head romaine lettuce, torn or chopped
- 1 small red onion, chopped
- 1 red bell pepper, chopped
- 1 cucumber, chopped
- 10 kalamata olives, pitted and sliced
- 1 dozen cherry tomatoes, halved
- 1/2 cup pecans, chopped, toasted lightly in dry iron frying pan
- 1/2 cup cranberries, dried

Instructions

- ☐ Mix together ingredients and toss with Creamy Salad Dressing (recipe on page 50).

Yam Orange Cups

Ingredients

- 4 yams, medium-size
- 4 oranges
- 2 oz. pecans, chopped, plus 8 whole pecans

Instructions

- ☐ Bake yams 1 hour at 350°F until tender.
- ☐ Cut oranges in half and scoop out insides.
- ☐ Place pulp in blender and blend slightly.
- ☐ When yams are cooked, scoop out insides and place in mixing bowl.
- ☐ Add pecans and 1 cup orange pulp and mash together.
- ☐ Fill orange halves with mixture, forming a round cone on top.
- ☐ With fork create circular texture and top each yam with 1 whole pecan.

Thanksgiving Veggie Turkey Roast

Ingredients

- 8 oz. cashew nuts, raw, whole and finely ground
- 4 oz. whole wheat bread-crumbs
- 1 egg, beaten
- 1 onion, small and finely
- chopped
- 2 cloves garlic, crushed
- 3 parsnips, medium-size, coarsely chopped
- 1 teaspoon rosemary, fresh, or 1/2 teaspoon dried
- 1 teaspoon thyme, fresh, or 1/2 teaspoon dried
- pinch of sage
- 1 teaspoon miso
- 1/2 cup water, hot
- 3 tablespoons olive oil
- 8 oz. mushrooms, chopped

Instructions

- ☐ Preheat oven to 350°F.
- ☐ Mix ground cashews with breadcrumbs. Add beaten egg to dry ingredients.
- ☐ In 1 tablespoon olive oil, sauté parsnips until soft and then mash.
- ☐ Mix parsnips and herbs into nut mixture.
- ☐ In 1 tablespoon olive oil, sauté onions with garlic until soft and add to mixture.
- ☐ Dissolve miso in 1/2 cup boiled water and add to mixture.
- ☐ In 1 tablespoon olive oil, sauté mushrooms, then add to mixture and mix all ingredients thoroughly.
- ☐ Grease baking tray with olive oil and shape mixture to look like turkey. Or to make a loaf, put mixture into olive oil–greased bread pan.
- ☐ Bake in oven for 1 hour covered, last 15 minutes uncovered.
- ☐ Serve with Mushroom Onion Gravy (recipe on page 51).

Breakfast Lunch **Dinner** Dessert Treats Beverages

Dessert Recipes

Breakfast Lunch Dinner **Dessert** Treats Beverages

Strawberry Tofu Cheesecake

Ingredients

- 2 lb. tofu, soft
- 1/4 cup olive oil
- 1/2 cup honey, unfiltered
- 1 tablespoon vanilla
- 1/4 teaspoon salt
- 2 tablespoons lemon juice
- 1 cup strawberries

Instructions

☐ Blend all ingredients (except strawberries) in blender.

☐ Pour the mixture into baked crust (recipe below).

☐ Bake for 30 to 40 minutes at 350°F.

☐ Let cool and then refrigerate.

☐ Before serving, slice strawberries or other fruit and arrange on top.

Crust for Strawberry/Tofu Cheesecake

Ingredients
- 1/2 cup cashews, whole
- 10 to 15 dates, pitted
- 1 tablespoon water

Instructions
- ☐ Preheat oven to 375°F.
- ☐ Chop cashews very fine in blender.
- ☐ Mix cashews and dates in food processor.
- ☐ Add up to 1 tablespoon water.
- ☐ Press mixture into baking pan. Bake for 4 to 5 minutes.

Contributed by Beatrix Rohlsen from *The Art of Taste*

Banana Ice Cream

To make this you will need a Champion juicer, or a single-gear Samson or Omega juicer. This can also be made in a blender with a jar attachment that screws into blade unit.

You will need to plan at least a day ahead of time.

Ingredients
- 1 ripe banana per person, peeled and frozen
- mango, berries, grapes, or other fruit, frozen

Instructions
- ☐ Put frozen bananas through the juicer (with special screen that contains no holes).
- ☐ Where the pulp usually comes out, your ice cream appears.
- ☐ Or place in blender jar and blend until smooth.
- ☐ Add frozen mango chunks, blueberries, grapes or strawberries.
- ☐ Mash together and serve immediately. This cannot be refrozen, as it will turn brown.

Melon Salad with Tahini Dressing

Ingredients
- 1 lb. ripe melon, cut in chunks
- 1 romaine lettuce leaf, shredded
- 1 tablespoon tahini, thinned with carrot juice or water

Instructions
- ☐ Mix together melon and shredded romaine and toss in Tahini Sauce (recipe on page 49).

Mango Strawberry Mousse

Ingredients
- 1 lb. tofu, soft
- 1 mango
- 2 tablespoons pure maple syrup
- 1 teaspoon vanilla
- 1 basket strawberries

Instructions
- ☐ Peel mango and cut off the meat.
- ☐ Put all ingredients except strawberries into the blender and puree until smooth.
- ☐ Pour into a bowl.
- ☐ Slice strawberries and mix into mango mousse.
- ☐ Cover with plastic wrap and refrigerate for at least 3 hours before serving.

Contributed by Beatrix Rohlsen from *The Art of Taste*

Baked Pears with Cinnamon

Ingredients
- 4 large pears, firm and ripe
- 1/2 teaspoon cardamom, ground
- 1/2 teaspoon cinnamon, ground
- 1/2 teaspoon cloves, ground
- 1 cup apple juice
- 1/2 organic lemon, organic and grate the rind

Instructions
- ☐ Peel pears and cut away cores.
- ☐ Cut in 1/2-inch slices and place in baking dish.
- ☐ Mix remaining ingredients and spoon over pears.
- ☐ Cover and bake at 350°F for 20 minutes.

Baked Apples with Raisins and Pecans

Ingredients
- 4 apples
- 1/3 cup orange juice
- 1/2 orange, organic and grate the rind
- 1/2 teaspoon mixed spices (cloves, nutmeg, cardamom)
- 1/4 cup raisins, unsulfured, soaked overnight
- 1/4 cup pecans, chopped

Instructions
- ☐ Peel top half of apples.
- ☐ Cut out stem end deeply and blossom end, slightly.
- ☐ Place in small casserole dish so apples fit well.
- ☐ Mix orange juice with orange rind and mixed spices.
- ☐ Add raisins and chopped pecans.
- ☐ Stuff center of apples where stem was removed, and pour the remainder in and around apples.
- ☐ Cover and bake at 350°F for 45 minutes or until apples are soft but not mushy.

Tofu Pumpkin Pie

Ingredients
- 1 1/2 packages tofu, extra-firm
- 15-oz. can of pumpkin puree
- 2/3 cup honey
- 1 teaspoon vanilla
- 2 teaspoons cinnamon, ground
- 3/4 teaspoon ginger, ground
- 1/4 teaspoon nutmeg, ground
- 1/4 teaspoon cloves, ground

Instructions
- ☐ Blend tofu in blender until smooth.
- ☐ Add remaining ingredients and blend well.
- ☐ Pour into Pie Crust (recipe below) and bake for about 1 hour at 400°F.
- ☐ Chill and serve. Filling will be soft, but will firm up as it chills.

Pie Crust for Tofu Pumpkin Pie

Ingredients
- 2 cups barley flour
- 1 cup oat flour
- 3 tablespoons olive oil
- 1/2 to 3/4 cup water

Instructions
- ☐ Mix grains and add olive oil. Add water to moisten. The dough should be as dry as possible to work with, to insure a softer crust.
- ☐ Prebake the pie crust in a 9-inch pie dish for 5 minutes at 450°F, before filling with Pumpkin Pie mixture (recipe above).

Nut Date Balls

Ingredients
- 1/2 cup cashews, raw and whole
- 1/2 almonds, raw
- 1/2 cup figs, dried and cut into small pieces
- 1 cup dates, cut into small pieces
- 1/2 cup coconut flakes
- *Optional: 1/4 cup brazil nuts*

Instructions
- ☐ Use food processor or blender to grind up nuts.
- ☐ Mush figs, dates and nuts together.
- ☐ Shape into little balls with wet hands and roll them in coconut flakes.

Contributed by Beatrix Rohlsen from *The Art of Taste*

Breakfast   Lunch   Dinner   Dessert   Treats   Beverages

Treats

Popcorn

Ingredients
- popcorn
- olive oil as needed
- yeast flakes to taste
- kelp powder, granulated, to taste

Instructions
☐ Popcorn is best air-popped.

☐ Sprinkle popped corn with olive oil, good-tasting yeast flakes, and granulated kelp powder or other creative spicy mixture! Yum!

Olive Oil Garlic Butter

Ingredients
- 1 cup olive oil
- 3 garlic cloves, crushed

Instructions
☐ Pour olive oil into short container.

☐ Add crushed garlic cloves and refrigerate.

☐ The oil becomes semi-hard and is easy to use as a spread.

Breakfast Lunch Dinner Dessert Treats Beverages

Apple Slices with Nut Butter

Ingredients
- 1 apple
- almond butter, sesame butter, or pure peanut butter

Instructions
- ☐ Slice apple and spread nut butter on slices.

Roasted Garbanzo Bean Nuts

Ingredients
- 1 can garbanzo beans (chick peas), cooked and rinsed
- 2 tablespoons olive oil
- 1 tablespoon lemon juice
- Sprinkle of cayenne pepper
- Sprinkle of sea salt

Instructions
- ☐ Toss cooked beans with remaining ingredients.
- ☐ Spread on a parchment-covered shallow baking pan and roast at 250°F for 50 minutes, stirring occasionally until beans are shrunken and brown

Breakfast Lunch Dinner Dessert Treats Beverages

Breakfast Lunch Dinner Dessert Treats Beverages

Corn Chips with Salsa or Guacamole

Ingredients
- 5 corn tortillas

Instructions
- ☐ Cut corn tortillas into pie-shaped slices.
- ☐ Place on cookie sheet and bake in oven at 250°F for 10 minutes.
- ☐ Remove and let cool and harden.

Salsa

Ingredients
- 2 ripe tomatoes, chopped
- 1/2 small onion, chopped
- small handful of cilantro, chopped
- 1 lemon, juiced
- *Optional: Guacamole (recipe on page xx)*

Instructions
- ☐ Mix together all ingredients and use as dip with home-made Corn Chips (recipe above) or raw vegetable sticks.

Almond Bread

Ingredients
- 1 lb. almonds, raw
- 2 eggs, beaten
- 1 1/2 teaspoons baking soda
- 1/2 teaspoon sea salt
- 1 tablespoon olive oil
- 3/4 cup water, carbonated

Instructions
☐ Preheat oven to 350°F. Blend almonds (a small amount at a time) in food processor or blender to fine texture.

☐ Place in bowl and add remaining ingredients.

☐ Pour into olive-oiled bread pan and bake 1 hour.

☐ Can stay fresh for over a week in an airtight container in refrigerator. Use for sandwiches or as a snack with Olive Oil Garlic Butter.

Fruit Juice Ice Pops

Ingredients
- 4 oranges, juiced, or 2 cups watermelon, blended

Instructions
☐ Use plastic ice pop molds or an ice cube tray and tooth-picks.

☐ Pour in juice and freeze.

Apple Jack Bread

Ingredients

- 1 lb. almonds, raw
- 2 eggs, beaten
- 1 1/2 teaspoons baking soda
- 1/2 teaspoon sea salt
- 1 tablespoon olive oil
- 3/4 cup water, carbonated
- 4 apples, peeled and chopped
- 1/2 cup raisins, unsulfured
- 1/2 cup walnuts, coarsely chopped
- 1/2 teaspoon cloves, ground

Instructions

☐ Preheat oven to 350°F. Blend almonds (a small amount at a time) in food processor or blender to fine texture.

☐ Place in bowl and add remaining ingredients.

☐ Pour into olive-oiled bread pan and bake 1 hour.

☐ Can stay fresh for over a week in an airtight container in refrigerator. Use for sandwiches or as a snack with Olive Oil Garlic Butter.

Breakfast   Lunch   Dinner   Dessert   Treats   Beverages

Beverages

kfast   Lunch   Dinner   Dessert   Treats   Beverages

Lemon Flush

Ingredients
- 1 large lemon or lime, peeled, seeded and cut into chunks
- 2 cups water
- pure maple syrup, or a few drops of liquid stevia sweetener
- sprinkle of cayenne pepper

Instructions
- ☐ In blender add lemon or lime plus 1/4 cup water and blend until liquid.
- ☐ Then add remaining water, 1 or 2 tablespoons maple syrup (to taste), and 1 to 3 shakes of cayenne pepper.
- ☐ Blend again and enjoy!
- ☐ This drink is great for the kidneys.

Almond Milk or Almond Banana Milk

Ingredients
- 1 lb. almonds, raw
- water as needed
- *Optional: ripe banana, cinnamon, nutmeg, or vanilla beans*

Instructions
- ☐ Grind almonds finely in food processor or blender.
- ☐ Slowly add water until a creamy consistency. Add other ingredients if desired.
- ☐ Strain in fine mesh strainer and store in refrigerator. (Mixture becomes thicker when stored so more water may need to be mixed in again when used.)

Iced Herb Tea

Ingredients
- Herbal tea bags, without caffeine
- 4 cups water
- Squeeze of lemon juice
- *Optional: raw honey or liquid stevia*

Instructions
- ☐ Choose a delicious herbal tea. Boil 1 cup of water.
- ☐ Place 3 to 4 tea bags in water for 10 minutes.
- ☐ Pour into pitcher and add 3 cups water and a squeeze of lemon juice.
- ☐ If sweetening is desired, add a little raw honey or a few drops of liquid stevia.
- ☐ Refrigerate before using.

Protein Smoothie

Ingredients
- 1 banana
- 1 cup vegetable juice, half carrot/half celery
- 1/2 cup strawberries, blueberries or peaches
- 2 tablespoons tahini

Instructions
- ☐ Blend until smooth.

Breakfast   Lunch   Dinner   Dessert   Treats

Beverages

Natural Soda Pop

Ingredients
- 1/2 cup fruit juice
- 1/2 cup sparkling water

Instructions
☐ Mix together and enjoy!

Rice Milk

Ingredients
- 4 cups water
- 1 cup brown rice, cooked
- 1 teaspoon vanilla extract
- 1 tablespoon pure maple syrup

Instructions
☐ Blend all ingredients together in a blender and then put through fine strainer. Refrigerate and shake before using.

Chapter 7
Questions and Answers

1. Are nuts and avocados too fattening to eat if I want to lose weight?

If you are doing a "weight loss" diet of only low-calorie foods, then nuts and avocados should be avoided. But low-calorie diets generally don't work. People feel hungry, deprived and resentful, then usually end up binging. It makes more sense to instead eat balanced healthful meals that contain a mixture of both low- and high-calorie foods. You may lose weight a little slower, but you will be developing a new way of eating that will transform your body to its healthiest state. Ultimately, healthful weight loss is easier to maintain by developing new eating habits, rather than going on periodic diets. Of course, if weight loss is your concern, it is best not to snack on or overeat nuts, avocados, desserts, or any other high-calorie foods. These foods should only be a portion of a balanced meal.

2. Will I ever be able to eat a chocolate bar or store-bought pizza again?

Of course, but it should be something only for special occasions. When you begin a healthier way of eating, it's important to stay away from "junk foods" for a while to help the body break old habits and learn new ones. After a month or two, having a small nibble once in a while should not disturb your progress. But be aware, sometimes a little taste can reawaken the addiction and it can take a lot of effort to free yourself again.

3. I have asthma, but if I stop eating cheese and milk, will I get enough calcium for my bones and teeth?

Absolutely. If you eat nuts and lots of green vegetables you get all the calcium you need. Dairy products contain cholesterol and can produce excess mucous in the respiratory tract and sinuses. This can contribute to asthma, allergies and stuffy noses, and therefore is not the best source for getting calcium. Actually, calcium-deficiency problems are caused more by things that drain calcium from the bones and body, than from the amount eaten. Some of these drains are soft drinks, coffee, aspirin and other drugs, and especially too much protein in the diet.

A good question to consider is, "Where do cows get all that calcium that ends up in their milk?" From eating grasses! Horses do the same. In fact, the largest land animal, the elephant, is a vegetarian — and it has those huge ivory tusks, made up of a lot of calcium!

4. If I only eat small quantities of meat or dairy, or even stop eating them all together, will I get enough protein?

New scientific evidence has shown that people of all ages actually need a lot less protein than was originally estimated years ago, and that all the food proteins we need are found in most foods. Of course, some foods have more quantities of protein than others. If your diet contains good quantities of beans, grains, nuts and vegetables, you will get all the protein your body needs — even enough for a growing kid. Remember that protein from animal sources comes with cholesterol and has no fiber. Also, laboratory experiments suggest that eating meat from animals that are given drugs, especially hormones to fatten them up, may contribute to cancer in humans. On top of that, most animals today are raised in miserable conditions, and eating meat supports that cruel treatment.

5. If I overeat healthy treats, can I get fat?

If you overdo anything, you may create problems…so the answer is yes. People usually know when they are overdoing something or "pigging out." For example, if you eat a large bowl of popcorn for an afternoon or evening snack, that should be fine. But if you have two or more bowls, that would be going overboard. The snacks in this book should be fine if they are eaten in the quantities suggested.

6. Do I need high-protein foods when I am sick with a cold or fever?

If you are ill, it is better to eat simple, easy-to-digest foods like fresh vegetable juices and blended vegetable soups. It is wise to stay away from the more complex foods until you are well. Resting is essential, and if you are resting, your calorie and protein needs are therefore much reduced. Also, during a cold it is important to eliminate all dairy and wheat products, since they can contribute to excess mucous.

7. Is all cholesterol bad for the body?

Small amounts of cholesterol are needed by the body to make certain hormones and for other uses. The body can actually produce all the cholesterol it needs from other fats (like fats from nuts and olive oil).

That means we do not need to eat animal products containing cholesterol to get what is needed by our cells.

8. I find it almost impossible to stay away from junk food. What can I do?

There are several reasons why people crave junk food. Sometimes it can simply be that people are not eating foods with enough vitamins and minerals in them, and the body therefore keeps craving more to eat. We usually translate that craving into junk food because it causes a quick reaction. Many times, when more high-nutrient foods are eaten, junk food cravings disappear. Of course, food can also be used to express emotional yearnings, in which case working with both a nutritionist and a psychologist or being in a support group for others that share this challenge, like Overeaters Anonymous, can be very helpful and supportive.

9. If I don't eat any animal products, do I risk a vitamin B12 deficiency?

There is still much controversy about vitamin B12. First of all, we actually need only a very small amount of this vitamin. Some scientists feel it is available only in animal products, while others feel it is in some seeds and vegetables, and is produced by bacteria in our lower intestine. Personally, I have never met a vegetarian with a B12 deficiency. The only people I've actually known who suffered from this problem had damage to the stomach cells that produce a substance called "Intrinsic Factor" that enables vitamin B12 to be absorbed into the body. This damage can happen through infections or from too much alcohol consumption. If there is doubt, it is easy to get a blood test checking vitamin B12 levels.

10. What if I start losing too much weight eating

more healthful foods?

Some people, especially children, burn calories very quickly and therefore need a higher caloric intake. In that case, I suggest increasing the quantities of foods eaten, especially extra amounts of nuts and avocados. Also, it's important to understand that when beginning to eat healthier foods, for the first month or two the body is cleaning out old stored toxins and clearing out unhealthy tissue and waste. This usually causes weight loss, even though food calories eaten are at normal levels. But after a few months, as the body rebuilds new tissue, there is a slow gain to the body's best weight, if that is needed. If there was too much weight to begin with, usually that weight will stay off as long as good food choices are maintained.

11. Should I take vitamins with this food program?

Meals containing a lot of vegetables, fruits, nuts and grains are packed with vitamins and minerals. Unless there is a problem with absorbing a particular nutrient, high-nutrient foods should provide all that is needed. Even with "so-called" depleted soils, plants won't grow unless the basic requirements of nutrients are available. Of course, organically grown food would be the best choice for highest nutrient levels without pesticide poisons. Rather than taking multi-vitamins and multi-minerals, specific supplements can be helpful for preventing or targeting certain conditions like arthritis, osteoporosis, digestive irritation, and heart disease. Certain antioxidants can help protect against cellular damage from environmental pollution. Advice from a knowledgeable nutritionist is the wisest way to determine what is needed.

12. I need caffeine to wake up in the morning. Is this harmful?

First thing in the morning, when the body is most sensitive, caffeine is a harsh jolt, which many people think gives them more energy. Actually, the opposite is true. Caffeine stimulates the body to burn its own energy faster, which feels like a rush of energy, but in fact is lowering our energy reserves at a time when they are already low from going six to eight hours without any food. That's why BREAKFAST is called that — because you are breaking the fast from the night before. First thing in the morning, having a freshly made vegetable juice or fruit, for example, actually gives the body a true burst of energy from the nutrient-rich foods that are quickly absorbed. That's the real thing!

13. If I want to be an athlete, shouldn't I eat lots of red meat?

You can get all of the necessary nutrients you need for strong muscles and high energy by eating meals high in vegetables, nuts, grains and beans, as well as eggs and fish if desired, but low in other animal products. There are many athletes, Olympic Gold Medal winners among them, who are even vegetarians. By the way, the strongest animals in the world are elephants, which eat only vegetable matter. That's true for gorillas, horses and cattle too.

14. Are eggs healthy to eat?

If the bulk of your food intake is high-fiber wholesome foods, occasional eggs should not create any problems since eggs can be good protein foods, even though they are rich in cholesterol. They also contain good amounts of a substance called lecithin, which actually helps to break down cholesterol. The important thing to know when choosing eggs is to buy them from chickens raised in a healthy or organic way — "free range" and without drugs. This means they are fed healthy chicken feed and are able to get exercise and sunshine. Most commercial chickens are instead locked into small overcrowded cages in dark factories and fed a lot of potentially dangerous hormones and drugs to over-stimulate egg production and to fight diseases that breed in these unnatural and cruel conditions.

15. What are the best oils to use on a salad, vegetables and popcorn?

All oils are high in calories. We love them because they dissolve flavor molecules in foods and make them more available to our taste buds, and the oily coating on food with oil on it allows for easier swallowing. Since oils digest slowly, they keep us feeling full longer. The healthiest oil to use is monounsaturated oil, which means it is more stable and less likely to become rancid at room temperature and when it's heated.

Polyunsaturated oils, like corn, safflower and peanut, are more unstable, meaning they could become rancid much easier and form free radicals, which may harm body cells. There are two monounsaturated oils on the market — olive oil and canola oil. Olive oil has been used healthfully over many centuries in the Mediterranean countries. Canola oil should be avoided since it is genetically engineered from toxic rapeseed oil. Some scientific studies indicate it may still contain low residues of toxic substances that could create long-term cellular damage. Olive oil should be cold-pressed or extra virgin and stored in glass, since oil can dissolve some of the polymers in plastic. Cold-pressed oil means It was pressed from the olive without using heat. Heat pressing produces more oil, but it destroys valuable vitamin E that occurs naturally in oil and protects the oil from becoming rancid. Since oil is high calories, and too much of it can put a strain on the gall bladder and liver, the daily healthful amount consumed should be around 2 oz. (4 tablespoons) daily, which should not be a problem, even if you are trying to lose weight.

16. Is margarine healthful to use since it has less calories than butter?

Even though margarine is made from vegetable oil, it is put through a process of hydrogenation (passing hydrogen gas through the oil), which changes its molecular structure to fats called "trans fats." Researchers believe trans fats, which have never been formed in nature before, may cause dangerous cell changes in the body after many years of use. Because of this, margarine should be avoided. Butter, on the other hand, is high in cholesterol and saturated fats, and therefore it should be used only sparingly, if at all. I suggest using olive oil instead, which becomes like a spread if you keep it in the fridge.

17. Can food affect my mood?

Most definitely, yes! Many children become hyperactive and lose the ability to concentrate after eating sugar and food laced with chemicals, like colorings. Sadly, many of these children are instead diagnosed with Attention Deficit Disorder and given strong drugs, when just getting them off junk food and increasing high-nutrient foods would help them be more balanced. Psychiatrists are now finding that many forms of mental illness improve with healthier dietary changes. Discover the effects for yourself. Pay attention to how you feel after eating different foods. Your own experience is the best way to learn. It is very important to understand that when someone starts to eat in a much healthier way, the body goes through a period of cleaning out. The skin may break out, and other cleansing actions may occur, especially moodiness, since old toxins and chemicals are being released by the organs and fat deposits, and cleaned out through the kidneys. As these chemicals are being flushed out, they can sometimes create a feeling of moodiness for a few days.

18. Are sugar-free foods made with artificial sweeteners good for weight loss?

Throughout the years, chemical sweeteners have been suspected of causing many problematic side effects — some very serious. For example, the sweetener aspartame, which is now listed under the natural flavor section and is found even in baby food, may be responsible for a wide range of health problems. When consumed, it is able to cross the blood-brain barrier, which can trigger serious reactions, including seizures and even death — as recently disclosed in Department of Health Service reports, which also list 90 different symptoms. The only sugar-free sweetener that appears to have no bad side effects is stevia, a natural food that in very small amounts is extremely sweet without the calories of sugar.

19. Does eating organic food really make a difference to my health?

All natural foods, such as fruits, vegetables, whole grains, nuts, and so on, are full of nutrients whether they are organic or not, though organic foods are generally higher in nutrients due to the way they are grown. Pesticides and chemicals in foods, such as preservatives and colorants, may be toxic to the cells, possibly causing serious disease later in life. Studies indicate this also may be so for non-organic dairy and animal products containing added hormones. Therefore, it makes sense to purchase organic foods when possible and avoid putting extra chemicals in the body. But if they are not available or too costly, I suggest peeling fruit and vegetables. As for lettuce and foods that can't be peeled, soaking them for 5 minutes in a pan of water with a capful of white vinegar or a vegetable wash product will help reduce any toxic residue on the surface.

It is important to be aware that harmful chemicals can get into your body from sources other than food. Toxic, harsh or irritating chemicals can be found in toothpaste, soaps, dish detergents, oven cleaners, floor polishes, hair products, household cleaners, nail polish and polish remover — even laundry detergent. We are fortunate that now it is possible to buy all these products in a healthier form from health food stores and even some supermarkets. Always read labels to find out the ingredients in products, and choose those with the least added chemicals — or better, no chemicals at all. Our precious bodies are worth it!

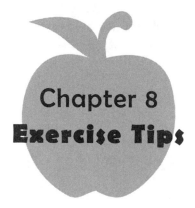

Chapter 8
Exercise Tips

Exercise is one of the major ingredients of staying in good shape, physically, healthwise, and mentally. Good exercise means stronger muscles, thicker bones, better circulation, and, for many people, a clearer mind.

An excellent exercise program is one that is consistent, at least three to five times per week. It's important to find a form of exercise that is enjoyable as well as being a good workout. If not, the mind will eventually rebel and create resistance to doing it. Exercising to music helps turn movement almost into a dance. Studying an Eastern form of exercise like karate, tai chi or yoga also helps to develop wisdom and awareness.

As important as exercise is, it is equally important to know when to rest. When feeling genuinely tired and sluggish, which is different from being lazy, or when having a cold or any illness, it is better not to exercise. Instead one should rest or nap. The reason is simple — there is not enough energy available in the body for exercise. It is being used someplace else in the body to do other work. Trust the body's wisdom. Listen to the body's message. If you go out and force exercise when you are not well, you may feel temporarily better, but you may have robbed energy from some other place and interrupted important repair work. Also if you push yourself and force energy back into the muscles, you are more likely to strain yourself at those times. Remember, the balance of exercise and rest is what serves health the most.

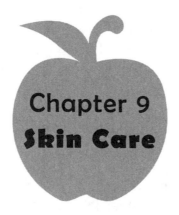

Chapter 9
Skin Care

Teenage skin problems have several causes, from over-production of oil glands, cleansing of the liver, higher levels of hormones, to emotional stress. The results of these actions, namely blemishes, can be minimized and in many cases eliminated by making a few changes.

Diet has a strong effect on the condition of the skin. Fried foods, fatty foods, chocolate and dairy products can aggravate skin problems and create excess skin oil. This is also true of heavily processed foods that are low in fiber, like pasta and cookies. They can lead to sluggish elimination, which slows down removal of waste from the body, creating a more toxic system, which in turn can contribute to blemishes.

On the other hand, foods with high-water and high-fiber content, like fruit and vegetables, flush the system. They allow the digestion to work quickly and efficiently, keeping the whole body clean. Vitamin A, which is found in carrots, yams, and other yellow and orange vegetables, and zinc, which is found in pumpkin seeds and grains, have been found to have beneficial healing effects on skin problems.

Keeping the surface of the skin clean of excess oil and bacteria build-up is also important. Washing the face morning and night with a mild non-soap cleanser and a good washcloth or natural sponge can work wonders. The texture of the cloth cleans deep down into the pores. Soaps and antibacterial cleaners can create an imbalance in the skin — stripping it of natural healthy bacteria, which actually protects the skin from problems. Also, although it is important to cleanse the excess surface oil with a mild cleanser and washcloth, it is important not to strip all of the skin's oil with harsh soaps, since a small amount of oil is protective and finer and purer than any moisturizer you could buy.

Emotional causes of skin problems are best dealt with by communication — expressing how we feel, letting others know what we need, and trying to understand how the people around us feel. Sometimes it is a good idea to talk with a school guidance counselor or psychologist who is there to help. Also, exercise may create a calming effect on strong emotions. If emotions are causing us continuous pain, they need to be paid attention to the same way we would pay attention to a pain in our stomach or any other place — by seeking professional help.

When it comes to caring for the skin, it is important to be aware of what is put on it. Skin medicines, makeup, creams and lotions many times contain chemicals that are not good for the body. When you put them on the skin, they seep into the cells. If you wouldn't want to eat it, then don't put it on your skin. Buy only products with pure and simple ingredients that won't in any way irritate or pollute the body.

A simple and healthy way to always have soft, moisturized skin, is to brush skin (arms, legs, back, chest, neck, feet) in the shower or bath with a medium strong natural bristle back brush. After the shower, massage a home-made oil mixture into the skin. To make this, put 1/2 cup each of avocado oil and almond oil into a dark glass bottle. Then add to the mixture the contents of 10 natural Vitamin E oil capsules (open capsules and squeeze out oil), plus a few drops of a scented essential oil that appeals to your sense of smell. Store in a dark, cool place. It will keep your skin beautiful.

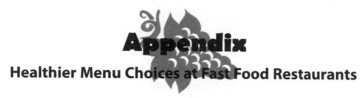

Appendix

Healthier Menu Choices at Fast Food Restaurants

Surprise – most fast food restaurants are now claiming to add healthier food choices to their menus. But are they really healthy - or are they still compromising quality for cheap ingredients?

Many of the fast food restaurants are advertising chicken salads and burgers without buns as healthier menu alternatives. The good thing about that is, by leaving out the bun many empty carbo calories that would turn into fat, are being eliminated. But problems still remain. Most of these restaurants are still cooking their chicken, burgers, fries and even fish in partically-hydroginated oils and fats – and that means you are eating TRANS-FATS! Shocking – especially after many newspaper articles and studies are showing that trans-fats may lead to heart disease and cancer.

Many people now order salads at fast food restaurants, thinking they are choosing a low calorie alternative – but most of the dressings on the salads contain some form of high-calorie sugar and/or clogging fat.

One of the bigger burger chains is now providing a veggie burger. The good news is that it has no artery clogging cholesterol – except for the mayonnaise and the bun that goes with it.

A popular Mexican fast-food restaurant is providing healthier items with their choice of toppings for tacos, and burritos. Instead of the usual high-cholesterol, high calorie cheese sauces, a tasty, much lower calorie but higher vitamin and mineral choice is a spicy tomato, onion veggie topping.

In all the 'new healthier' fast food choices I saw, sadly, many still contained some unhealthful ingredients that were cheaper then using a healthier product. The bottom line – you must read the ingredients! Most fast food restaurants have flyers you can request which describes each ingredient in every menu item.

Be good to your body - make informed choices!

Suggested Reading

For more tasty, easy-to-make, nutritious recipes, I suggest the following cookbooks:

Barbara Cousins, *Cooking Without*, Thorsons/HarperCollins Publishers, 2000.

Alan Goldhamer, *The Health Promoting Cookbook: Simple, Guilt-FreeVegetarian Recipes*, Book Publishing Company, 1997.

Mary and John McDougall, M.D., *The New McDougall Cookbook*, Plume/Penguin Books, 1997.

Beatrix Rohlsen, *The Art of Taste*, Gourmet Creations Publishing, 1994.

If you are interested in reading more about the body/food connection, I strongly suggest:

Joel Fuhrman, *Disease-Proof Your Children*, St. Martin's Press, 2005.

Douglas J. Lisle and Alan Goldhamer, *The Pleasure Trap: Mastering the Hidden Force that Undermines Health and Happiness*, Healthy Living Publications, 2003.

John Robbins, *Diet for a New America*, H. J. Kramer, reprint edition, 1998.

Excellent books for healing chronic digestive problems:

Kendall Conrad, *Eat Well, Feel Well*, Clarkson Potter Publishing, 2006.

Elaine Gottshall, *Breaking the Vicious Cycle*, Kirkland Press, 2004.

To find out if there is a health risk with any product you are using, or to discover healthier products available:

Debra Lynn Dadd, *Home Safe Home: Protecting Yourself and Your Family from Everyday Toxins and Harmful Household Products*, Jeremy Tarcher/Putnam, 1997.

Debra Lynn Dadd, Judy Collins, and Steve Lett, *Nontoxic, Natural and Earthwise*, Houghton Mifflin, 1990.

Other works by Dale Figtree:

Dale Figtree, Ph.D., *Health after Cancer*, Hanuman Press, 1985.

Dale Figtree, Ph.D., *The Joy of Nutrition* (video), produced by Win Win Productions, 2003.

Index of Recipes

Freshly Made Juices

Breakfast Recipes

Lunch Recipes

Salads

Dressings and Sauces

Dips, Spreads, and Pita Pockets

Dinner Recipes

Main Courses

Soups

Holiday Dinner Menu

Desserts

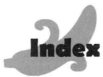

Index